COMPLEMENTARY CURES

More than 530 "Blended Prescriptions"
for Healing Dozens
of Common Conditions—
Better and Faster

By the Editors of *Prevention* Health Books

RODALE

ST. MARTIN'S
PAPERBACKS

Prevention's Best is a trademark and *Prevention* Health Books is a registered trademark of Rodale Inc.

COMPLEMENTARY CURES

© 2000 by Rodale Inc.

Book designer: Keith Biery
Cover designer: Anne Twomey

ISBN 0–312–97480–9   paperback

Printed in the United States of America

Rodale/St. Martin's Paperbacks edition published May 2000

St. Martin's Paperbacks are published by St. Martin's Press, 175 Fifth Avenue, New York, NY 10010.

10 9 8 7 6 5 4 3 2 1

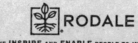

RODALE

WE INSPIRE AND ENABLE PEOPLE TO IMPROVE
THEIR LIVES AND THE WORLD AROUND THEM

Notice

This book is intended as a reference volume only, not as a medical manual. The information given here is designed to help you make informed decisions about your health. It is not intended as a substitute for any treatment that may have been prescribed by your doctor. If you suspect that you have a medical problem, we urge you to seek competent medical help.

This book was developed with the assistance of David Edelberg, M.D., assistant professor of medicine at Rush Medical College in Chicago and chairman and founder of the American WholeHealth Centers in Chicago, Boston, Denver, and Bethesda, Maryland.

Contents

Preface

The future of health care can be found in a nondescript office tower in a bustling neighborhood of Chicago. It is here, at American WholeHealth Centers, that David Edelberg, M.D., and his fellow healers are practicing a bold new form of medicine.

Doctors, acupuncturists, nutritionists, Chinese medicine experts, herbalists, and massage therapists all share space—and patients. Their premise is simple: provide people with the best healing solutions that exist. If that happens to be a prescription drug, so be it. But sometimes, it might be an herb. Or acupuncture treatments. Or a nutritional makeover. Sometimes, it just means listening to the patient for as long as it takes. Most likely, it is a combination of many things, most—if not all—of them natural, simple, and time-tested.

Underlying their work is an important realization: While conventional medicine—that is, everyday, American-style, Dr. Welby medicine—is uniquely powerful at dealing with things like heart attacks, injuries, and major bodily breakdowns, it is not the best healing method for much of what ails people. This is an opinion that more and more health care consumers share. Yet the health care industry is slow to respond.

Fortunately, there are rays of light breaking through these clouds. Around the country, independent clinics similar to American WholeHealth Centers are being established. They combine a world of healing practices in ways that truly optimize the curing process. And they will continue to emerge. Why? Because their solutions work.

We call this new approach blended medicine. Its premise is that by taking the best solutions from many healing disciplines and doing them in combination, you absolutely maximize your potential for healing and health.

The "blended prescriptions" this approach produces are what make this book so unique, so powerful. We have taken several dozen of the most common health problems and put together blended prescriptions for each.

To do this, we interviewed as many natural, alternative, and conventional health practitioners as we could to get their favorite solutions. We then asked Dr. Edelberg and his staff at American WholeHealth Centers to help us prioritize these solutions and formulate specific remedy plans. The result is blended prescriptions for each problem, plus a slew of other alternatives that you might wish to consider as well.

Of course, as with any medicinal remedies, these prescriptions can have side effects. Please read the precautions in Using Self-Care Safely on page 253 before treating yourself.

We are extremely grateful to Dr. Edelberg and his staff for all their time and help in shaping the solutions presented inside. We believe these are some of the most potent healing prescriptions ever put to the page. Use them and consider yourself at the forefront of health care. It will feel better than you could possibly imagine.

Blended Medicine: A New Approach to Health Care

There's a Velvet Revolution going on in the healing world: Masses of Americans are seeking out and using alternative medical treatments. From herbal medicine to massage, from homeopathy to meditation, alternative modalities are increasingly welcome in American homes.

News of the uprising came in the early 1990s, when the *New England Journal of Medicine* published an eyebrow-raising report on just how many Americans were using alternative medicine.

One in three of those surveyed said that they had used at least one unconventional therapy in the past year. That works out to an estimated 60 million adults.

Two-thirds of those who took advantage of alternative medicine did so on their own, the report found, without seeing a professional. But the report also concluded that Americans in 1990 visited alternative medicine providers 425 million times. That's more than the 388 million visits they made to conventional primary care physicians.

No better indication of the popularity of alternative medicine exists than the shifting attitude of the medical establishment. Historically, conventional medicine tended to either ignore alternative medicine or scoff at it. Now, the *Journal of the American Medical Association* is publishing peer-reviewed articles on alternative topics, and some managed-care organizations are offering alternative therapies as an "expanded benefit." Blue Cross even uses its new coverage of some alternative treatments as a selling point.

Medical education is adjusting, too. Institutions such as Bastyr University in Seattle offer rigorous programs in natural medicine, producing not M.D.'s but N.D.'s, naturopathic doctors, who use natural agents such as food, plants, water, and exercise to assist the body in healing disease and promoting wellness. And alternative principles, especially mind-body theories, may finally be gaining a toehold in established medical schools. "It certainly has become respectable to talk about these things at the highest academic level," says Larry Dossey, M.D., former chief of staff at Medical City Dallas Hospital; author of several books, including *Healing Words: The Power of Prayer and the Practice of Medicine*; and executive editor of the medical journal *Alternative Therapies*. "They are becoming part of the curriculum."

Physicians who integrate unconventional methods into their practices report that other doctors are sending more patients to them for alternative treatments. "Colleagues are referring patients to me regularly now," says Alan Brauer, M.D., who uses alternative modalities in his practice at TotalCare Medical Center in Palo Alto, California. "Thirty years ago, nobody would. That's fairly amazing."

The People's Choice

Why the surge in interest? Here are some of the reasons that have been suggested.

You want more options. If something is not getting the job done, it is logical to try something else. "For acute illness—from myocardial infarctions to broken bones—conventional medicine is very effective," Dr. Brauer says. "But conventional medicine is not effective for many other kinds of health issues."

You know it works. When a group of medical researchers in Oregon polled family practice patients about why they had also chosen to make use of alternative medicine, the answer was straightforward. "The main reason was a belief that it would work," the researchers write in the *Archives of Family Medicine.*

You want alternatives. Alternative medicine shines where conventional medicine is weakest—in dealing with chronic ailments such as back problems, depression, and pain that won't go away, explains Dr. Dossey. And with today's longer life spans, there's inevitably more chronic disease, notes Dr. Brauer. So people are looking at alternatives more often.

You want control. Access to alternative treatments means you can try various options and decide what is right for you. Furthermore, most alternative modalities insist that you become informed about the "whys" of any treatment and participate actively in it. Unlike many conventional physicians, alternative practitioners want you to assume control. "Educating patients is a distinguishing factor in alternative treatment," says C. Norman Shealy, M.D., Ph.D., founding president of the American Holistic Medical Association and director of the Shealy Institute for Comprehensive Health Care in Springfield, Missouri.

You prefer natural remedies if possible. Yes, technology has worked wonders in medicine. "But it has become unbearable for patients," says Christina Stemmler, M.D., who practices Western and Chinese medicine and is the director of the Center for Integrated Medicine in Houston. "They are the ones who experience the side effects of prescription drugs, of surgical interventions, of hospital stays, when an herb or acupuncture needles are all they need."

You care about prevention. The spirit of the times emphasizes prevention of illness. Alternative medicine is

Some Light on the Blind Spots

The typical physician sees the human body as basically a complex machine, with disease being a breakdown of parts. This has brought many great advances in Western medicine. But the approach is incomplete. As we learn the strengths of other forms of medical practice, it becomes apparent that conventional medicine has a number of blind spots.

It underplays self-healing. Modern medicine's tendency to "nuke" disease often does little to promote self-healing.

It underemphasizes prevention. "We're too busy taking care of disease to try to prevent it," observes C. Norman Shealy, M.D., Ph.D., founding president of the American Holistic Medical Association and director of the Shealy Institute for Comprehensive Health Care in Springfield, Missouri.

It neglects nutrition. Medical journals are loaded with information about the role of nutrition in health. Medical practice isn't. "Go to a hospital and look at the meal trays that the patients get," says Christina Stemmler, M.D., who practices Western and Chinese medicine and is the director of the Center for Integrated Medicine in Houston.

It keeps the mind and body too far apart. Although mind-body unity is gradually gaining acceptance, most of the available techniques are largely ignored in favor of clearly in the lead here. Conventional medicine cares about prevention, of course, but more in theory than in practice, according to David Edelberg, M.D., assistant professor of medicine at Rush Medical College in Chicago

what conventional doctors believe really does the job—the surgical operation or the prescription.

It is too specialized. Patients today may find themselves shuttling among several different specialists, each treating different ailments or body parts.

It has lost the personal touch. The personal touch that disappeared along with the house call was more than just a nicety. "When the old family doctor came to your home, he put his hands on you, and that was perhaps the most healing thing he had to offer," Dr. Shealy notes.

It has lost touch, period. Even the most conservative medical schools require courses on the "healing partnership" between patient and doctor. "But that disappears under the weight of all the emphasis that's placed on technological interventions," says James S. Gordon, M.D., clinical professor in the departments of psychiatry and community and family medicine at the Georgetown University School of Medicine in Washington, D.C. "And physicians aren't trained to listen to patients in an open way. They are trained to listen only for clues as to what they should do."

It mixes the sick with the well. The conventional system is very good for very sick people, but not so good for the general population. "It uses the same technology on the well as on the sick—and sickens the well," Dr. Stemmler says.

and chairman and founder of the American WholeHealth Centers in Chicago, Boston, Denver, and Bethesda, Maryland. "Conventional physicians are concerned with diagnosis—CAT scans, MRIs—and with therapies like chemo or radiation," he says, "but not a whole lot with prevention."

What Health Really Means

Alternative therapies can be defined as medical interventions that are neither taught widely in U.S. medical schools nor generally available in U.S. hospitals. A few of them are homeopathy, naturopathy, traditional medicines from China and India, biofeedback and other mind-body processes, acupuncture, aromatherapy, and body-oriented treatments such as massage or Rolfing.

But what is it that ties together these seemingly disparate approaches to medicine?

"The alternative view is that health is a continuum ranging from poor to excellent," Dr. Brauer says. "You can be in poor health without having a disease. And optimum health is more than just the absence of disease."

"The concept of disease is what essentially separates the two kinds of medicine," says Leo Galland, M.D., a physician in New York City who is director of the Foundation for Integrated Medicine and author of *Power Healing*. "Western medicine will ask what disease the person has and then treat that disease. But my approach is to try to understand all the factors that are contributing to sickness in all dimensions and what can be done to correct them."

In other words, while conventional medicine attempts to fight disease, alternative practitioners see their task as a broader one: to maintain (or restore) a healthy balance.

"In all alternative healing systems, including all ancient and traditional healing systems, sickness is perceived as the result of disharmony or imbalance," Dr. Galland says. "The role of the healer is to identify what those imbalances are and help the individual to correct them." The aim is not to defeat disease but to encourage the body's natural healing system.

"Alternative modalities share the philosophy that symptoms are part of the body's attempt at self-healing," says Jennifer Jacobs, M.D., a homeopathic physician, assistant clinical professor of epidemiology at the University of Washington in Edmonds, and coauthor of *Healing with Homeopathy*. "Rather than trying to take away the symptoms, we try to strengthen the overall system so that the body is better able to heal itself."

The Energy of Living

Encouraging self-healing and restoring balance are pretty much the same thing in alternative medicine. And both are related to a subtler concept that's universal in alternative medicine but missing in conventional Western medicine.

This concept sees the entire interplay of an individual's health and happiness as being linked in an energy system or vital force. There are upward of 50 names for this energy flow, but you will mostly hear the Chinese version *chi* or *qi* (both pronounced "chee").

"Virtually all fields of alternative medicine regard disease as the end stage of energetic imbalances," Dr. Edelberg says. "Disease in these areas of healing comes about when mind issues and body issues have produced an imbalance of energy, affecting an organ by depletion or stagnation of the energy."

Interestingly, this concept that is so foreign to conventional medicine's way of thinking is the theoretical basis for an alternative modality that has gained perhaps the most acceptance by standard medicine: acupuncture.

Because the Chinese were able to map the chi flow through the body, they discovered that needles temporarily inserted at strategic points could (probably via electromagnetic impulses) unblock energy or otherwise correct imbalances in its flow. The therapeutic value of acupuncture is wide, from pain relief and addiction treatment to relief of menstrual or menopausal symptoms, explains Dr. Stemmler.

Tapping the Power of Nature

Alternative treatments have a lot in common on the practical level as well. A good example is their emphasis on the natural. Whether they use herbs, music, aroma, body work, or mind-body techniques, alternative practitioners shun drugs or invasive surgery unless it is absolutely necessary.

"I've seldom used antibiotics, and everybody has gotten well," says William Mitchell, N.D., a naturopathic physician and cofounder of Bastyr University in Seattle. "It's not that I have a problem if an antibiotic is indicated. But the vital force is pretty amazing, and it just turns out that in most cases it is up to the task with the use of natural medicines."

Herbs, of course, are the quintessential natural medicine, and they are used as healing tools worldwide. But there are other ways to take advantage of the plant world's therapeutic riches. One with implications for personal wellness strategies is aromatherapy, in which the essential aromatic oils of herbs are inhaled or applied to the skin with the hope of therapeutic benefits.

Putting Alternative to the Test

"No matter what alternative therapy we are talking about, we have the obligation to furnish proof that it works," says Larry Dossey, M.D., former chief of staff at Medical City Dallas Hospital, author of several books, and executive editor of the medical journal *Alternative Therapies*.

The worry is that analyzing alternative medicine by using conventional testing methods amounts to forcing square pegs into round holes. The roundest hole is standard medicine's double-blind controlled clinical trial. "If you use only randomized clinical trials, some alternative methods can be tested," Dr. Dossey says. "Herbal medications can be tested, like any other medication, but other alternatives can't."

Making clear the official position, Wayne B. Jonas, M.D., director of the Office of Alternative Medicine at the National Institutes of Health (NIH) in Bethesda, Maryland, says, "Not only can complementary and alternative medicines be examined using the same criteria as in professional Western medicine, they must be."

Indeed, acupuncture may seem an unlikely alternative candidate to pass conventional muster, but pass it did. The NIH itself put together a panel of experts to evaluate the existing research, and the conclusion was that acupuncture "is an effective treatment for nausea caused by cancer chemotherapy drugs, surgical anesthesia, and pregnancy and for pain resulting from surgery and a variety of musculoskeletal conditions."

"The important thing to remember is that there are thousands of ways to test," Dr. Dossey says. "You don't always have to spend millions of dollars to get good evidence that something works."

If *natural* is a word that ties together the alternative practices, so is *holistic*. It might more usefully be spelled "wholistic" because it refers to the alternative practitioner's preference to treat the whole person—mind, body, and soul. It also means dealing with the whole health picture, not just sharpshooting symptoms.

You can get a good idea of how this works by looking at the headache. A conventional physician typically will do two things: First, he'll relieve the symptoms with some kind of painkiller. Second, he'll make sure that it is not something serious like a brain tumor. This can be done in a 5-minute office visit. "The holistic perspective, however, regards the headache as yet another sign of the wisdom of the body," Dr. Edelberg says. "It's alerting you that something is amiss." The range of things that might be amiss is so wide that nothing but holism could deal with it. Maybe your computer is positioned at the wrong height. Or your typical lunch of a doughnut and diet cola is catching up with you. Or your boss is a jerk. Or the carpeting fumes are nauseating.

"Healing comes about by making the appropriate lifestyle change," Dr. Edelberg says. "Suppressing the headache with an over-the-counter medicine misses the point. It's like taking the phone off the hook when someone is calling to let you know that your house is on fire."

The Power of Listening

How do alternative practitioners get at all these factors? "It's simply a matter of spending time with people," says James S. Gordon, M.D., clinical professor in the departments of psychiatry and community and family medicine at the Georgetown University School of Medicine in Washington, D.C. "As physicians, we should be concerned about what you are concerned about. Your arthritis, for example, may persist because of ways that you are stuck in your life, stuck in your diet, stuck in your exercise habits, stuck in your attitude."

Listening helps with more than diagnosis, says Dr. Gordon. "The relationship between doctor and patient is the fundamental part of the treatment. The most important thing is my helping that person figure out how to move ahead in life. So I'm not only listening for symptoms to treat but also seeing what that person can do for himself."

Is this a new breakthrough in medicine? Only if you consider something 5,000 years old as new. That's how long traditional Indian medicine, a star player on the alternative roster, has been diagnosing people by a time-consuming process of observing them, questioning them, touching them, and taking their pulses. Known as Ayurveda, Indian medicine uses natural remedies such as herbs, oil, and steam, but it puts major emphasis on lifestyle adjustments. So does traditional Chinese medicine, often abbreviated in English as TCM. Also thousands of years old, TCM has lots of techniques at its disposal—acupuncture, acupressure, Chinese herbs, and massage being just some of them—which it uses in a very sophisticated, systematic way. Like Ayurveda, however, it stresses diagnosis arrived at through patient but thorough personal observation and communication.

Multiplying Your Options

The most exciting prognosis for the new century has nothing to do with the latest miracle-drug-of-the-month coming out of the medical labs. It has everything to do with time-honored alternative healing methods finally taking their rightful place alongside standard medicine as legitimate remedies and effective ways to prevent disease.

Indeed, the very term *alternative* is moving aside for the more inclusive word *integrative*. That's because it is no longer a question of either staying with conventional medicine or turning to alternative modes. It is a question of integrating both into an expanded vision of healing. You can blend the approaches to get better results.

That could mean trying, say, homeopathic remedies to help your body heal itself instead of resorting to a drug. It could mean taking advantage of healing herbs while you use conventional symptom relievers. Or it could mean convalescing more quickly and comfortably with alternative techniques after conventional medicine has done its thing.

And, of course, it can mean taking the strictly conventional route if that's the best choice for what ails you. Best of all, it can mean blending alternative-inspired prevention strategies—such as a pro-health diet, vitamins, stress reduction, and social/spiritual engagement—with other good modern health practices to keep yourself balanced and disease-free.

The point is that your healing options today are infinitely greater than they were yesterday. Alternative medicine has brought to the party its cornucopia of natural remedies, time-honored therapies, innovative techniques, and holistic approaches. So not only do you now have more options, you have more combinations of options that you can use to find the healing strategies that are right for you. And you will find them in this book.

A Nation of Blenders

Actually, the odds are pretty good that you are already taking advantage of blended medicine. The same research that tells us one-third of adult Americans use alternative medicine also reveals that four out of five of those alternative-medicine users seek conventional treatment at the same time. We are already becoming a nation of blenders.

Stealth Blending

When it comes to blending alternative treatment with conventional medicine, a lot of folks pursue a "don't ask, don't tell" policy. Their doctors don't ask them if they are also using alternative remedies, and patients don't tell them if they do. A full 7 out of 10 people using alternative medicine fail to inform their physicians about it, according to David Eisenberg, M.D., director for the Center for Alternative Medicine Research at the Beth Israel Deaconess Medical Center in Boston.

The truth is, it's in your best interests to let your doctor know what other remedies you are taking or therapies you are undergoing. Safety is a major reason; some remedies just don't go together. Effectiveness is another; if you are sneaking back and forth, you may be working against yourself. You may not be using the combination of systems in the optimum way.

And as any married couple knows, keeping secrets weakens a relationship. "The delivery of medical care, like the experience of illness, is best viewed as a journey shared," says Dr. Eisenberg.

This trend is growing as more and more conventional M.D.'s are converting to an integrated practice. The result is an increasing number of clinics and medical centers that put the best of alternative and conventional medicine under one roof. Many of the medical experts that you have been hearing from in this book run clinics that are typical of the new availability of integrated medicine.

For example, Dr. Edelberg's American WholeHealth clinics employ conventionally trained but alternative-experienced physicians to offer a rich mix of internal medicine, family practice, acupuncture, behavioral counseling, and relaxation techniques. Dr. Stemmler blends traditional Chinese medicine with the conventional Western variety, which means that acupuncture and Chinese herbs are standard treatments in her family practice. Dr. Gordon is the founding director of the Center for Mind-Body Medicine in Washington, D.C., which promotes the integration of mind-body healing techniques with conventional medicine. And that is exactly what he does in his own medicine and psychiatry practice, in which he includes relaxation therapies, hypnosis, meditation, acupuncture, nutrition, musculoskeletal manipulation, and physical exercise.

These, of course, are just a handful of integrated medicine clinics nationwide. Add to them the plethora of qualified homeopaths, naturopaths, and trained herbalists and acupuncturists, among many others, and you get an idea of the healing opportunities that are out there. But it is the M.D.'s with integrated practices who best symbolize the new medicine.

"A true integrated or blended practitioner isn't biased," Dr. Brauer says. "I try to keep one foot in conventional medicine and one foot in alternative medicine. In the middle is the blended area. So I'm equally likely to pre-scribe an antibiotic as an herbal remedy."

What it all comes down to is that the appeal of blended medicine for a doctor (who wants to heal) is the same as it is for you (who want to be healed). "It puts two tool-boxes at our disposal: conventional and alternative," Dr. Edelberg says. "I for one could never return to the limited approach of using only conventional medicine."

What's New at the Drugstore

While it's not always easy to find an integrative physi-cian or alternative practitioner, much of the medicine they use is a lot easier to get these days. Putting the home remedies offered in this book to use usually requires little more than a trip to your local drugstore or health food store.

"The products are much more available, and that is ab-solutely a good thing," Dr. Brauer says. "The field is moving toward greater openness, which means more pos-sibilities for health."

Homeopathic remedies, for example, have found their way out of the homeopaths' offices and onto retail shelves. Medicinal herbs in easy-to-use pill and tincture forms are being sold by many companies, bringing price and quality competition to the field, to the benefit of customers.

Even more available than the remedies is information about them. The Internet is the prime mover in this in-formation boom, of course, but it's certainly not the only source of knowledge, as browsing in a major bookstore, a magazine rack, or a video catalog will confirm.

There are a few things to keep in mind when choosing an alternative cure. For one, information overload is cre-ating for alternative medicine the same conflicts that have plagued conventional medicine—one research team's miracle remedy is another's toxic pariah. And the sheer volume of available remedies invites misuse by the careless or foolhardy.

All in all, though, what blended medicine can do for your self-care is just what the doctor ordered, so to speak. "There has never been a better time for self-healing than today," Dr. Brauer says. "There's more interest; there's more availability of products; there's vastly more information."

A Matter of Comfort

Why is the future of blended medicine so bright? Because the way we think about it has changed. Not only do we find the therapies useful, but the very idea of alternative medicine has become comfortable. As Dr. Edelberg puts it, "With so much of the population using alternative medicine regularly, there is no longer the need to demystify it that there was just 5 years ago."

That shouldn't be surprising. After all, conventional and alternative medicine have the same goal: to promote health. The practitioners may use different tools and approaches, but they are essentially doing the same thing, which is using knowledge and experience to heal. Enlarge your perspective a little, and you may find that the two may be more alike than not.

For example, is taking an herb in capsule form all that different from swallowing a prescription drug? Remember, pharmacological research for drug development often begins with medicinal plants. And herbs can provide the model, or even the basic materials, for drug synthesis. When primitive medicine men prescribed tea from willow bark, they were taking advantage of the same active ingredient that's in aspirin.

The overlap makes it a lot easier for newcomers to accept alternative medicine. The shift in thinking is not always that radical. Nutritional therapy? Hey, our moms clued us in to that early on. Relaxation therapy? You don't have to convince us that we feel better when we are not uptight. Extended diagnostic interviews? All along we wanted to be listened to. Holism? It is no secret to us that we are more than a collection of organs.

So it is not a case of alternative being from Venus and conventional from Mars. They are both very much of this Earth. And together, they are a powerful healing team.

Acne

Just beneath the surface of your skin, the sebaceous glands rooted in your dermis secrete an oily, waxy substance called sebum. When all goes well, sebum travels smoothly up the hair follicle and escapes through pore openings to the skin's surface. When all doesn't go well, those same hair follicle cells churn out a fibrous protein called keratin at an alarming rate. This keratin is the stuff that can create a major roadblock inside your pores.

When keratin gets in the way, sebum becomes trapped beneath your skin, along with dirt and menacing bacteria. As a result, your hair follicle swells or even ruptures. And a pimple rears its ugly head.

The Blended Prescription

Note: To learn about cautions and possible side effects of the remedies in this chapter, see page 253.

You can take quick action to help banish acne the moment it appears, but a healthy diet is the key to long-term prevention. Try to eat as many fruits and vegetables as possible and clear out all junk food, especially the kinds that are high in saturated fat. Avoid red meat, fried foods, margarine, milk, and other milk products. And stay away from food products that contain hydrogenated vegetable oils. That done, here is a six-step prescription for short- and long-term relief from acne, created by our panel of blended-medicine experts.

Wash with glycerin soap two or three times a day. It is gentle and very good at getting rid of excess oil.

Wash with a 5 percent solution of benzoyl peroxide, following the package instructions.

Drink two to three cups of burdock (*Arctium lappa*) tea, red clover (*Trifolium pratense*) tea, or both every day.

HERBAL POWER

The Tea Tree Solution

To kill acne-causing bacteria on contact, arm yourself with a facial soap that contains tea tree (*Melaleuca alternifolia*) oil. This strong therapeutic oil harbors abundant antiseptic, antibacterial, and anti-fungal properties, and it is considered a strong acne fighter, says Jennifer Brett, N.D., a naturopathic physician in Norwalk and Stratford, Connecticut. Diluted tea tree oil solutions also are available for skin application.

Steep 1 tablespoon of the herb in one cup of boiling water for 5 to 10 minutes; then strain before drinking. These teas flush the liver of toxins and boost immunity.

Take your vitamins. Several vitamins are crucial to skin health and may help prevent outbreaks of acne.

Vitamin A: 100,000 international units (IU) every day for 2 weeks, then reduce the dosage to 25,000 IU daily

Vitamin E: 400 IU twice a day

B vitamins: B-complex 50 twice a day

Vitamin C: 1,000 milligrams three times a day

Mix 1 tablespoon of flaxseed (*Linum usitatissimum*) oil with food or juice and take it every day. Flaxseed oil has been shown to help many skin conditions, including acne.

Drink 2 tablespoons of borage (*Borago officinalis*) oil each morning. Borage oil helps with the production of prostaglandins that reduce inflammation.

Other Approaches

Add evening primrose (*Oenothera biennis*) oil to your diet. In addition to the 1 tablespoon of flaxseed oil in the

blended prescription, take 1 tablespoon of evening primrose oil a day, says David Edelberg, M.D., assistant professor of medicine at Rush Medical College in Chicago
and chairman and founder of the American WholeHealth
Centers in Chicago, Boston, Denver, and Bethesda, Maryland. Flaxseed oil, containing alpha-linolenic acid, is a
natural source of omega-3 fatty acids. Evening primrose oil
contains gamma-linolenic acid and is high in omega-6
fatty acids. Taken together, they can clear up acne by reducing inflammation, pain, and swelling.

**Take a homeopathic remedy that is tailored to your
type of acne.** If your acne is chronic, painful, itchy, contains pus, and produces superficial scarring, take Sulfur,
recommends Sujatha Pillai, a homeopathic physician at
American WholeHealth Centers in Chicago. If your acne
tends to form cysts and leave deep scars, and it is very
painful and slow to heal, Silicea may be the right choice,
Pillai says. Graphites is also available if your acne often
exudes pus and forms a crusty coating. You can take each
homeopathic remedy daily until your acne clears up.

Start with either a 6C or 12C strength in pill form,
following the label directions. If you have a flare-up after
2 to 3 days, be patient—it means the remedy is working.
If there isn't any change after 7 days, however, stop that
potency and start taking 30C, repeating the previous
steps.

**When nothing else works, see your doctor about pre-
scription medication.** If you develop severe acne that
doesn't respond to over-the-counter medications or natural remedies, a dermatologist can prescribe topical and
oral antibiotics that are very effective in reducing the bacterial growth that can cause acne. Consider tretinoin
(Retin-A), a vitamin A derivative, if you have mild to
moderate acne. Or consider isotretinoin (Accutane), the
strongest oral acne medication available.

Arthritis

Arthritis is easily recognized by its most unwelcome calling card: achy chronic joint pain and swelling that leads to limited movement and stiffness. While there are more than 100 forms of this disease, osteoarthritis is by far the most common. It's wear and tear at its worst—with the cartilage that cushions your joints degenerating faster than it can be rebuilt.

The Blended Prescription

Note: To learn about cautions and possible side effects of the remedies in this chapter, see page 253.

Doctors often recommend over-the-counter or prescription medications that are classified as nonsteroidal anti-inflammatory drugs (NSAIDs) for relief from arthritis. But there is concern that these drugs can actually deter joint tissue from rebuilding. Fortunately, you can effectively relieve arthritis pain and ease inflammation by using natural remedies. Here are seven approaches that help give quick as well as long-term relief, as prescribed by our blended-medicine experts.

When pain is severe, apply ice; when stiffness is severe, apply heat. A clever ice-treatment approach is to freeze water in a paper cup, peel the sides down, and massage the joint with the exposed ice. Apply the ice directly to the skin, and keep the ice moving to prevent it from freezing your skin. Do this for 15 to 20 minutes, three or four times a day, until the pain and swelling reduce. As for heat, apply a heating pad no more than 15 minutes at a time, three or four times a day.

Rub capsaicin ointment into painful joints three times a day. Use over-the-counter brands such as Capzasin-P or ArthriCare Ultra Rub.

HERBAL POWER

Nine in a Joint Venture

Certain herbs can be very beneficial to joint health, says Glenn S. Rothfeld, M.D., clinical assistant professor at Tufts University School of Medicine in Boston and author of *Natural Medicine for Arthritis*. He recommends a mixture of nine herbs: white willow (*Salix*, various species) and stinging nettle (*Urtica dioica*) for their anti-inflammatory effect; calendula (*Calendula officinalis*) and white peony (*Paeonia lactiflora*) for their ability to detoxify joints; horsetail (*Equisetum arvense*) to strengthen connective tissue; and rosemary (*Rosmarinus officinalis*), yarrow (*Achillea millefolium*), juniper berries (*Juniperus*, various species), and cornflower (*Centaurea cyanus*) for their overall antirheumatic effect.

Combine equal amounts of each dry herb in a large jar or other airtight container. Use 1 heaping teaspoon per cup of boiling water. Let the tea steep for 15 minutes to reach a healing strength. Strain, then drink two to three cups a day, says Dr. Rothfeld.

Take two tablets of acetaminophen every 4 hours to relieve pain. Avoid NSAIDs like ibuprofen and naproxen, however, except for occasional relief. They may aggravate certain preexisting gastrointestinal conditions such as ulcers and inflammatory bowel disease.

Supplement with 500 milligrams of glucosamine sulfate three times daily—and give it time to act. Glucosamine is a naturally occurring chemical found in joints that stimulates connective-tissue repair and new cartilage growth. It also reduces pain and inflammation. Keep in mind, though, that it may take about 6 weeks before you start getting pain relief from it. If you get stomach irritation, reduce the dose.

Be sure to take the following five nutritional supplements. The three vitamins help prevent tissue damage, while the two minerals rebuild cartilage.

Vitamin A: 5,000 international units (IU) per day

Vitamin E: 400 IU per day

Vitamin C: 3,000 milligrams per day

Zinc picolinate: 30 milligrams per day

Copper: 2 milligrams per day

For a homeopathic remedy, try Rhus tox. 6C or Bryonia 6C. For either remedy, take two pellets every 15 minutes for four doses, then two pellets every hour for four doses on the first day. After that, take two pellets every 6 hours for 2 to 3 weeks.

Rub arnica (*Arnica montana*) ointment on painful muscles as often as needed.

Other Approaches

Lift some light weights. An interesting new way to treat arthritis takes the focus off the joints and strengthens the surrounding muscles instead, says Glenn S. Rothfeld, M.D., clinical assistant professor at Tufts University School of Medicine in Boston and author of *Natural Medicine for Arthritis.* "Gentle weight training makes a lot of sense for arthritis," he says. Stronger muscles at either end of an arthritic joint mean that the cartilage in between won't have to work as hard—and that means less pain.

Seek out food suspects with an elimination diet. For about one-third of all people with arthritis, sensitivity to one or more foods may be to blame for the pain, says John Irwin, M.D., a retired gynecologist from Litchfield, Connecticut, and author of *Arthritis Begone!* Eliminating those

SKILLFUL HEALERS

Apitherapy

Would anyone in his right mind ever ask for a bee sting? How about 20 of them? If you sought out the care of an apitherapist, that is precisely what you would be doing. Apitherapy, the medicinal use of bee venom and other bee products, has been practiced since the time of the ancient Greeks, and today it's practiced by more than 10,000 Americans.

Bee venom contains anti-inflammatory substances that can relieve arthritis, according to Glenn S. Rothfeld, M.D., clinical assistant professor at Tufts University School of Medicine in Boston and author of *Natural Medicine for Arthritis.*

You will need to see a qualified apitherapist, a person who has been trained to use bees and their products for treating disease. The American Apitherapy Society (AAS) can provide a list of practitioners judged by their review board to have excellent training and skill. Contact the AAS by writing to them at 5370 Carmel Road, Hillsboro, OH 45133.

The apitherapist uses tweezers to hold the bee and control stinging. Then he applies the bee to the area it is supposed to sting, either directly on the sore joint or in a trigger point.

The number of stings and the duration of the treatment depend on you and your arthritis. If your condition is ongoing and troublesome, you might require several stings at a time, two or three times a week, for up to 3 months.

foods, which aren't the same for all food-sensitive people, can mean an improvement in both pain and swelling.

To discover if your arthritis is related to a food sensitivity, Dr. Irwin recommends that you follow the Class One diet for 1 week. This basic, limited diet is designed to rule out your most common trouble foods. If you are one of the people affected by food, this step alone will most likely give you some blessed—and quick—pain relief, according to Dr. Irwin.

In the Class One diet, the safe foods to eat are limited to the following:

- Fruits: Avocados, grapes, olives, peaches, pears, plums, and prunes
- Vegetables: Cauliflower, celery, lettuce, olives, parsley flakes, peas, spinach, and winter squash
- Starch: Rice
- Oils: Olive oil
- Fish: Cod, flounder, salmon, trout, and tuna
- Water and salt as needed

If you experience significant relief on the Class One diet, you can start identifying which trigger foods you need to avoid. Reintroduce potential trouble foods into your diet one at a time. Those foods can include anything that is not in the basic diet, such as bananas, lamb, shellfish, dairy products, and caffeine. After you have reintroduced the food, eat a good amount of it during the next day or two. If you have no reaction, then you can add that food to the "friendly" list. But if arthritic symptoms flare up, mark down that food as a troublemaker.

Drop the trouble food from your diet forever, then wait until you are feeling painless again before you resume your food sleuthing. In time, you will have a range of safe foods to choose from and a list of pain-producing foods to avoid.

This dieting should be safe for everyone, but people who have diabetes or are on other special diets should check with their doctors before trying it.

Back Pain

Your back is a large expanse of muscles, nerves, tendons, and numerous other elements—all supported on an array of intricately sculpted bones called the vertebrae. Given the complexity of this setup, it is no wonder that pain can radiate from many sources. If you lift a heavy box without bending your knees or if you jump out of bed too quickly, you may tense a back muscle so quickly that it goes into a spasm, sending out one kind of pain signal. Then tissues become inflamed, which makes even more of your nerves scream for mercy.

Another potential source of pain is the vertebrae themselves. The lower-back, or lumbar, disks are particularly susceptible because that is where most of your weight rests when you're sitting.

Finally, emotional stress as well as physical stress can complicate the pain picture.

Most of us will experience a bout of back pain at least once in our lifetimes, if not more often. When you do, it is likely that you will feel better long before you discover why your back hurts in the first place.

The Blended Prescription

Note: To learn about cautions and possible side effects of the remedies in this chapter, see page 253.

Though you may be tempted to collapse into bed at the first sign of back pain, many experts say that you should resist that temptation. Depending on what is triggering your pain, inactivity may actually lengthen your recovery time. So rather than resting passively, take steps to help yourself in other ways. See your doctor if your back pain persists for longer than a week, if it worsens with time, or if it is accompanied by a fever.

Here is how to put together your own seven-step treatment for acute back pain, as prescribed by our blended-medicine experts.

Immediately take an over-the-counter anti-inflammatory medication such as ibuprofen, following the instructions on the package. Or take 750 milligrams of the supplement bromelain at a potency of 2,400 mcu (a standard unit of measurement for enzymes) three or four times a day between meals, gradually reducing the amount needed to control the pain. This pineapple-based enzyme is effective at reducing pain and inflammation, but it takes less of a toll on your stomach than some of the popular over-the-counter anti-inflammatories.

Get into a shower and aim the comfortably hot water at the painful area of your back. Gently bend forward, then left and right. Bend carefully to the point of pain and, if you can, an inch or two farther. Do this a total of 10 times in each direction. This should help relax the muscle.

After the shower, massage the painful area with arnica (*Arnica montana*) oil or Traumed ointment. Look for both in a health food store. (Traumed products also are available from your health care provider under the name Traumeel.) Arnica relieves pain and has anti-inflammatory properties. Traumed ointment contains a combination of homeopathic ingredients.

In addition to their topical forms, take two tablets of the homeopathic medicine Arnica 6C every hour or take Traumed tablets, following the directions on the package.

SKILLFUL HEALERS

Chiropractic

Chiropractors do hands-on manipulation to help treat back pain. In addition, they often treat these problems with devices that generate mild electrical currents. Treatment with electrical stimulation helps disperse swelling, calm painful nerve endings, and speed healing of injured tissues. Electrical stimulation is particularly useful when back pain has you frozen into position or when you feel so sore that you don't want anyone to touch you, according to Joseph Smith, D.C., a chiropractor with Chiropractic Associates in Fogelsville, Pennsylvania.

Use visualization to help with the pain. Imagine that there is a knot in your back and you are slowly loosening that knot.

Drink an herbal tea to relax your muscles. Try any of the following: hops (*Humulus lupulus*), valerian (*Valeriana officinalis*), passionflower (*Passiflora incarnata*), or skullcap (*Scutellaria lateriflora*). You can also take these herbs as tinctures. Use 30 to 45 drops to one cup of water.

If pain persists, ask your doctor about a prescription muscle relaxant such as cyclobenzaprine hydrochloride (Flexeril) and, if necessary, a stronger painkiller such as acetaminophen (Tylenol) with codeine or ketorolac tromethamine (Toradol).

Other Approaches

Use an "emergency" acupressure point to relieve acute back spasms. Just below your nose, centered above your upper lip, is a slightly concave area called the philtrum.

This is the point called Governing Vessel 26, says Efrem Korngold, O.M.D., a doctor of Oriental medicine and licensed acupuncturist at Chinese Medicine Works in San Francisco. This point stimulates what Chinese medicine calls a meridian (a channel through which the body's motivating energy flows) that bisects the top of the head and runs along the length of the spine to the tailbone.

"You will want to use your thumb to press up into that notch rather hard, causing a sensation of soreness," says Dr. Korngold. Press into the point with your thumb for about a minute or until you feel the spasm abate. You can repeat this procedure every 10 to 15 minutes as needed.

To help strengthen your back and prevent future injury, make it a habit not to sit all day long. Your back is much better off when you are standing upright because you put an enormous amount of pressure on the lumbar disks when you are sitting down, according to Joseph Smith, D.C., a chiropractor with Chiropractic Associates in Fogelsville, Pennsylvania. And that lumbar pressure is even worse if you slouch forward in your seat.

To help withstand the strain, stand whenever you are talking on the phone or answering your mail and lean back occasionally to stretch your back, advises Dr. Smith. Combined with good posture, that will give your lower back the relief it needs.

Breathe slowly and deeply to lower your stress level. "I see three types of stressors, in particular, that affect the lower back: fear, anger, and financial problems," says Dale Anderson, M.D., clinical assistant professor at the University of Minnesota Medical School in Minneapolis and author of *Muscle Pain Relief in 90 Seconds: The Fold and Hold Method.* Whenever you feel the tension that accompanies stress, begin a slow deep-breathing exercise, he advises. Sit in a comfortable position and expel as much breath as possible through your mouth. Then, breathing in through your nose as you fill your lungs with air, let your diaphragm (located in your upper abdomen) expand. If you can maintain this deep breathing with a simple, slow in-out rhythm, counting as you go, you can relieve the tension.

Begin a daily abdomen-strengthening workout. Abdominal exercises can do a lot to protect your back, says Andrew T. Weil, M.D., clinical professor of internal medicine and director of the integrative medicine program at the University of Arizona College of Medicine in Tucson and author of *Spontaneous Healing*. "They are a good antidote to back pain because they balance and tone the muscles that support the spine."

Try three sets of basic stomach crunches every day to add some strength and support to your midsection. Lie down on your back on a carpeted floor or exercise mat with your knees bent at a 45-degree angle and your feet flat on the floor about hip-width apart. Place your palms on top of your thighs. Keeping your chin lifted and your eyes on the ceiling, slowly curl your upper body toward your knees so that your shoulders lift a few inches off the floor. Hold that position a moment, then lower your shoulders and repeat. Try to do 10 repetitions.

Bad Breath

Bad breath can be caused by your lunch or dinner menu, alcoholic drinks, cigars, cigarettes, or certain notorious foods like garlic and onions. But the underlying cause of obnoxious breath is bacteria that thrive in an oxygen-deprived environment. These so-called anaerobic bacteria can live almost anywhere in your mouth—in the crevices between your teeth or the tucked-in nether regions of your tongue—announcing their presence with fumes that hitch a free ride on the warm, moist breeze of your breath.

The Blended Prescription

Note: To learn about cautions and possible side effects of the remedies in this chapter, see page 253.

Visit your doctor if you think that your bad breath may be related to other health problems. (Chronic breath odor can sometimes be caused by gum disease, sinus infections, diabetes, or kidney trouble.) Then use these five approaches from our team of blended-medicine experts to chase out the bad odor.

Just before bedtime, floss, brush, and scrape your tongue from back to front—in that order—to beat the odor-causing bacteria that thrive at night. You can pick up a flexible tongue scraper along with floss and toothpaste at the drugstore.

Drink lots of water throughout the day to keep your mouth moist, hydrate your whole body, and help avoid morning breath. Drink eight 8-ounce glasses daily.

To counteract breath odor, place a drop or two of essential oil of peppermint (*Mentha piperita*) directly on your tongue.

Carry along some cloves or aniseeds to chew when you need them. One clove likely will do the trick; two or three aniseeds are about the right dose.

Check your local drugstore for a supplement that contains parsley seed oil. Breath Assure, which is just one of the products made with parsley seed oil, can help eliminate temporary bad breath that comes from garlic, coffee, or onions, says Anthony Dailley, D.D.S., founder of the Center for Breath Treatment in San Francisco.

Bladder Infections

Normal urine flow begins with your kidneys. These purplish brown organs remove liquid waste—urine—from your blood. The urine flows down narrow tubes called ureters into the bladder. Acting like a big water tower, the bladder stores the urine until it is time to empty it out of the body through the urethra.

Bladder infections often result when bacteria from a different neighborhood, usually from the colon, decide to take up residence near the opening of your urethra. These out-of-towners have sticky, hairlike structures that help them muscle their way onto the walls of your urethra.

From there, the bacteria migrate to your bladder, where they quickly establish a home. The burning sensation you may feel while urinating is due to the acid in the urine that washes across the irritated urethra walls, which are rubbed raw by bacteria.

The Blended Prescription

Note: To learn about cautions and possible side effects of the remedies in this chapter, see page 253.

See a doctor immediately if the burning sensations are accompanied by a persistent fever for more than 24 hours or if you feel lower-back pain, which signals that the bladder infection is spreading to your kidneys. In such cases, you will receive antibiotics or antibacterial drugs to stop the spread of infection. For less-troublesome cases, here is a four-step prescription from our blended-medicine experts to eradicate the bacteria and bring relief to your bladder. If it doesn't make a difference in 2 days, see a doctor.

Drink lots of water. You know you are getting enough water when your urine is colorless. The goal is to constantly flush the bad bacteria out of your bladder and urethra.

HERBAL POWER

A Soothing Tea

For lasting relief against many bladder infection symptoms, try this herbal tea blend created by Jill Stansbury, N.D., a naturopathic physician in Battle Ground, Washington, and assistant professor and chairman of the botanical medicine department at the National College of Naturopathic Medicine in Portland, Oregon. Combine 1 ounce of pipsissewa leaf (*Chimaphila umbellata*), 1 ounce of marshmallow root (*Althaea officinalis*), ½ ounce of pot marigold flowers (*Calendula officinalis*), and 1 ounce of chamomile flowers (*Matricaria recutita*). Put 1 tablespoon of this mixture into one cup of boiling water. Steep it for 20 minutes, then strain and drink.

Consume up to five cups of this herbal tea each day until the symptoms disappear. "This is an antibiotic alternative for simple infections," says Dr. Stansbury.

In addition, drink six glasses of unsweetened cranberry juice every day. Sweeten it with a little honey if it is too tart for you. Or take two 100-milligram cranberry extract capsules every 2 hours for 8 hours, tapering off to four two-capsule doses per day. Cranberry prevents bacteria from sticking to the bladder wall and causing infection.

Start with 2,000 milligrams of vitamin C, then take 1,000 milligrams every 4 hours while you're awake. This will bolster your body's attack on the infection.

If those steps seem to be working after 2 days, continue the two capsules of cranberry extract four times a day and reduce the dosage of 1,000 milligrams of vitamin C to three times a day, for at least 7 days.

Drink the herbal teas marshmallow (*Althaea officinalis*), chamomile (*Matricaria recutita*), and echinacea

(*Echinacea purpurea*) with goldenseal (*Hydrastis canadensis*). These herbs possess a slew of soothing and healing properties. Echinacea is an immune system booster, goldenseal fights infection, marshmallow soothes the burning, and chamomile calms inflammation.

Other Approaches

If the doctor puts you on a prescription of antibiotics, follow up by taking two capsules of acidophilus twice daily for 2 months. Antibiotics wipe out some good bacteria as well as bad, and the supplement acidophilus helps restore the balance of beneficial bacteria in your urinary tract, says Mark Stengler, N.D., a naturopathic physician in Carlsbad, California, and author of *The Natural Physician*. "Acidophilus acts like a bodyguard. It protects against infection and helps prevent an overgrowth of bad bacteria," he says. Check the label carefully: Your daily dose should contain a minimum of one billion active cells.

Skip the jalapeños and spicy salsa. Eating any type of spicy food will only prolong your bladder infection by aggravating the inflammation. "Hot, spicy foods go into the area of infection and only make it hotter," says David Molony, Ph.D., executive director of the American Association of Oriental Medicine and a licensed acupuncturist in Catasauqua, Pennsylvania.

Stay away from foods high in acid or sugar, which can trigger or worsen bladder infections. Oranges, limes, lemons, grapefruit, and tomatoes can irritate the bladder wall, and sugar can stymie healing. All should be avoided until the infection has disappeared, says Dr. Stengler.

Bronchitis

When a pesky virus or bacteria get into the lungs, the bronchial tubes respond by swelling and filling with mucus. As the tubes thicken, the tiny airways become even tinier, and soon you have uncontrollable spells of coughing and hacking, your body's way of clearing out the mucus. Along with that come "special gifts" of the bacteria or virus, like soreness in the chest and back, sore throat, fever, fatigue, breathlessness, and the chills.

The Blended Prescription

Note: To learn about cautions and possible side effects of the remedies in this chapter, see page 253.

Bacterial bronchitis demands special attention that you may not need for viral bronchitis, so the first step is to visit a doctor and determine which form of the bug you have. If it is bacterial, your doctor will prescribe antibiotics. If it is viral, you may still receive antibiotics to prevent secondary bacterial lung infections, like pneumonia, that can take advantage of your weakened condition.

Tried-and-true cold remedies may be the best treatment for bronchitis's similar symptoms. So drink lots of water and tea, use a vaporizer, stay home from work, and rest.

Use those conventional treatments in tandem with the following five natural medicines for a speedier recovery, say our blended-medicine experts.

Give yourself a dose of 50,000 international units (IU) of beta-carotene three times a day and 2,000 milligrams of vitamin C three times a day. These supplements give your immune system the boost it needs to battle the infection.

In addition, take 200 milligrams of echinacea (*Echinacea purpurea* or *Echinacea angustifolia*)—with or

without the same amount of goldenseal (*Hydrastis canadensis*)—four times a day for 1 week. These herbs also bolster immunity.

To help thin mucus, take two 375-milligram capsules of bromelain at a potency of 2,400 mcu (a standard unit of measurement for enzymes) three times a day between meals. Bromelain is an enzyme from pineapple that breaks down mucus.

Use eucalyptus (*Eucalyptus globulus*) essential oil as a chest rub. Dilute two drops of the oil in 1 ounce of almond

---

HERBAL POWER

A Balm for Bronchitis

The medicinal herbs that are commonly used for colds, influenza, and sinusitis can also be used to speed recovery from bronchitis, says Ellen Evert Hopman, a master herbalist in Amherst, Massachusetts; a professional member of the American Herbalists Guild; and author of *Tree Medicine, Tree Magic*. Following is an herbal tea recipe brimming with antiviral and antibacterial compounds to help break up lung-clogging mucus, suppress coughing, build immunity, and scoot you along to a speedy recovery, she says.

Place 6 cups of water in a nonaluminum pot. Add 2 teaspoons each of mullein (*Verbascum thapsus*), astragalus (*Astragalus membranaceus*), balm of gilead (*Populus candicans*), bayberry bark (*Myrica cerifera*), apple tree bark (*Pyrus malus*), and fresh ginger. Cover the pot tightly. Let the herbs simmer for 20 minutes. Strain into a cup and drink, says Hopman.

As an alternative, you might find a ready-made "bronchitis tea" with these or other herbal ingredients in a health food store.

oil or castor oil before you rub it liberally on your chest. Cover the oiled area with plastic wrap, then a thin towel, and apply a heating pad to help the oil penetrate your tissues.

For a soothing steam inhalation, put a few drops of eucalyptus oil in a pan of water and heat to boiling. Then remove the water from the stove and inhale the steam safely but deeply.

Other Approaches

Have hot, healing drinks to clear your mucus. If you have white mucus, slice a piece of fresh ginger into three or four slivers about ¼ inch thick. Put them in a small pot, add 2 cups of water, cover, and simmer for 20 minutes. Strain the ginger tea into a cup and add honey and lemon to taste. Drink up to one cup of this brew two times a day. In Chinese medicine, ginger is known to work like a detergent, sweeping white mucus from your throat, explains David J. Nickel, O.M.D., a doctor of Oriental medicine and licensed acupuncturist in Santa Monica, California. But be warned that it has the opposite effect if your phlegm is yellow, he adds.

Kelp works as a cleanser on yellow phlegm, explains William D. Nelson, N.D., a naturopathic physician in Colorado Springs, Colorado. Add ½ teaspoon of powdered kelp to one cup of hot water and drink it as a tea once a day. Or if you don't like the concentrated taste of sea vegetables, add ½ teaspoon of kelp powder to strong-tasting soups or use it to "salt" your meals throughout the day, he suggests.

Consider cough syrup. If natural remedies don't seem to be working, you may do better with an over-the-counter cough syrup such as the standard Robitussin syrup, or Robitussin-DM for severe coughing. Follow the package instructions. These are very effective at dealing with the

SKILLFUL HEALERS

Reflexology

If a bout of bronchitis has laid you low, reflexologists will tell you that some foot treatment may be just what you need to get on your feet again. A reflexologist's fingers will stimulate the reflex areas on your feet that correspond to your adrenal glands. This treatment can reduce bronchial tube, nasal, and sinus inflammation, says Laura Norman, a licensed massage therapist, a leading reflexology authority in New York City, and author of *Feet First: A Guide to Foot Reflexology*.

In addition to providing treatments that home in on your diaphragm, chest, and lung regions, helping to break up congestion, the reflexologist may work on your toes to unblock energy flow circulating through your shoulders, head, and neck. This helps open up sinus and nasal cavities, she says. You may also get treatment in the part of the foot designated as the spleen area to help build resistance and speed the elimination of toxins from your body.

symptoms of bronchitis, but be aware that they do nothing to solve the underlying problem and may cause some side effects.

To soothe your chest and stimulate healing, blend four essential oils. Using a base of 1 ounce of olive oil or sweet almond oil, add two drops of Roman chamomile (*Chamaemelum nobile*), one drop of hyssop (*Hyssopus officinalis*), two drops of lavender (*Lavandula officinalis*), and five drops of eucalyptus (*Eucalyptus globulus*), suggests Ixchel Leigh, an aromatherapist and regional director of the

National Association for Holistic Aromatherapy in Durango, Colorado. Rub the mixture liberally on your chest and upper back, Leigh suggests.

Apply acupressure to the rim of your ear. Place your index finger inside the most concave part of your outer ear, directly across from your ear canal. Now place your thumb directly behind the ear, opposite the finger. This is your lung point, according to Dr. Nickel. Squeeze firmly as you exhale for 5 seconds. Loosen your grasp, then inhale for 5 seconds. "You will increase oxygen and blood circulation in the infected area, reduce pain, and encourage easier breathing," he says. You should feel relief in 1 to 2 minutes.

Squeeze the adrenal point on your ear. By applying pressure to another part of your ear, "you will stimulate your adrenal gland to produce cortisone, which is the body's natural pain reliever and anti-inflammatory hormone," says Dr. Nickel. Grasp the fleshy piece of cartilage that covers your ear opening and pinch it firmly between your thumb and index finger while you exhale through your mouth for 5 seconds. Loosen your grip and inhale for 5 seconds. Repeat for 2 minutes.

Take Aconitum napellus 30C if you have symptoms caused by cold, dry air. If you have been out in the cold and find yourself wheezing and coughing with severe congestion, this homeopathic remedy may relieve your symptoms, says Kristy Fassler, N.D., a naturopathic physician in Portsmouth, New Hampshire. Take three pellets twice a day for 2 days.

Use the homeopathic medicines Antimonium tartaricum 6C or Arsenicum album 6C. Take two pellets every 15 minutes for four doses, then two pellets every hour for four doses on the first day. If your symptoms persist, take two pellets four times a day until the symptoms resolve.

Bruises

Picture spilled soda seeping under a glass tabletop, and you have the idea of what happens whenever you knock your body hard.

Bruises are collections of blood in the tissues right under your skin. At the point of contact, small capillaries break open, releasing blood. The swelling you may experience is actually a result of the protective nature of your small blood vessels, which form clots or squeeze down to prevent further bleeding.

Busy working round-the-clock, your white blood cells will recover this blood and deliver it to your lymphatic system, which reabsorbs and recycles it back into the bloodstream. This reabsorption of aging, spilled blood creates a visible rainbow effect on your skin.

The Blended Prescription

Note: To learn about cautions and possible side effects of the remedies in this chapter, see page 253.

"Over time, 99 percent of bruises get back to the point where there is no evidence of ever having a bruise," says John McCabe, M.D., professor of emergency medicine at the State University of New York Health Science Center at Syracuse. That said, see a doctor if you develop unexplained bruises or if one seems significantly larger than the injury warrants. But for the typical bruise, here is a program for fast healing and pain relief from our blended-medicine panel.

If it's available, immediately apply essential oil of lavender (*Lavandula*, various species) or witch hazel to the bruise. Lavender helps lessen the flow of pain impulses. And witch hazel contains tannins, natural astringents that help shrink swollen and inflamed tissue.

SKILLFUL HEALERS

Acupuncture

Once your doctor has ruled out serious injury, acupuncture can quickly reduce redness, swelling, and pain associated with bruises, says Mark Michaud, M.D., a family physician with American WholeHealth Centers in Chicago. If you are new to acupuncture, expect the visit to last about 30 minutes, he says. Although needles may be inserted around the borders of the bruise, you should experience little or no pain. The needles stimulate the release of endorphins, the body's feel-good hormones, and they relieve blockage of the body's natural energy flow to the site, explains Dr. Michaud.

Wrap a cold pack in a cloth or towel and hold it on the bruised area for 5 minutes. Apply it twice an hour, for just 5 minutes, during the first day or two. The cold will help reduce swelling.

After each cold-pack application, spread on arnica (*Arnica montana*) ointment or Traumed ointment. Look for Traumed products in a health food store. They are available from health care providers under the name Traumeel. Arnica relieves pain and has antiseptic and anti-inflammatory properties. Traumed ointment contains a combination of homeopathic ingredients.

To promote fast healing, take two pellets of Arnica 6C, a homeopathic remedy, every 15 minutes for four doses. After that, take two pellets every hour for four doses, then every 6 hours until your symptoms disappear. Or use the tablet or liquid form of the homeopathic remedy Traumed, following the package directions.

For pain, take Arnica 6C as described above or two tablets of acetaminophen every 4 hours as needed. Don't take aspirin or medicines containing ibuprofen. These and other nonsteroidal anti-inflammatory drugs (NSAIDs) inhibit the action of blood platelets that are needed to stop beneath-the-skin bleeding.

Pick up some Bach Rescue Remedy at your health food store and follow the instructions on the label. This multipurpose flower-essence remedy is known for its comforting and soothing effects.

Other Approaches

Take 1,000 milligrams of vitamin C three times a day, 400 international units (IU) of vitamin E once a day, and 10,000 IU of vitamin A twice a day. This vitamin trio helps your skin heal and helps build collagen, the high-protein fiber that is your skin's foundation, says Mark Michaud, M.D., a family physician with American WholeHealth Centers in Chicago. It also helps strengthen capillary walls, he adds.

Take 500 milligrams of bromelain at a potency of 2,400 mcu (a standard unit of measurement for enzymes) three times a day between meals. Bromelain contains a protein-digesting enzyme that works to decrease inflammation in the bruised area, says Mark Stengler, N.D., a naturopathic physician in Carlsbad, California, and author of *The Natural Physician*.

Apply bruise plaster when you sleep at night. This tarlike substance can be found in Chinese drugstores and large Chinese grocery stores, according to David Winston, a founding professional member of the American Herbalists Guild and founder and president of Herbalist and Alchemist in Broadway, New Jersey. "It's like tar spread on a flexible cloth. You unroll it, and it sticks on bruises. Use it overnight, and the next morning, your bruise will look more like it is 3 weeks old." The plaster helps move stagnant blood out of the bruised area, he says.

Burns

Skin shields your body against infection and dehydration, but it provides little protection when you scorch yourself with an iron, get a searing sunburn, or spill a boiling liquid on it.

With the mildest burns, the outer layer (called the epidermis) and the uppermost part of the dermis redden and swell. Moderate burns dig deeper into the second layer of skin, the dermis, which houses blood vessels, lymph vessels, nerves, and hair follicles. These burns often cause blood vessels to leak blood serum into the inflamed area, causing the two skin layers to swell and separate, resulting in blisters. At the same time, nerve endings get stretched, which creates a pain sensation.

The most severe burns bore down through the dermis to the subcutaneous fat layer. With these burns, the skin is charred black or a grayish white, and it actually feels waxy or leathery to the touch. Severe burns also destroy nerve endings, so the burned area is numb rather than in pain.

The Blended Prescription

Note: To learn about cautions and possible side effects of the remedies in this chapter, see page 253.

If your burn is so severe that the skin is grayish and numb, you should get to an M.D. or the emergency room right away. Also see a doctor if you have blistery burns over a skin area wider than your fist or if these burns are on your face, hands, feet, groin area, or buttocks.

As long as you don't have the kind of severe burn that requires emergency treatment, cool water, in the first step below, is your first and best ally simply because it stops the heat from spreading. Then try the six other steps from our blended-medicine experts to help relieve pain, prevent scarring, and facilitate healing.

Run cool water over the burned area as soon as possible. Or apply a cold compress—a cold pack, a bag of ice, or even a bag of frozen vegetables—wrapped in a towel.

When the skin temperature normalizes, pat the area dry with a clean, soft cloth. Then apply an aloe vera gel or cream, essential oil of lavender (*Lavandula*, various species), or silver sulfadiazene (Silvadene) cream, available by prescription, to help soothe and heal the skin. To figure out if your skin temperature is back to normal, do a touch test: Gently rest your fingertips on the burned area and then on the normal skin nearby. If the burned area feels hotter than the normal skin, it needs more cooling.

For the pain, take aspirin, acetaminophen, or ibuprofen as directed on the bottles. Or take two pellets of Arnica 6C, a homeopathic remedy, every 15 minutes until you get relief.

Use vitamin E cream at any time during the healing process to prevent scarring. Or open a vitamin E capsule and spread the oil over the burn. Burns cause the body to produce more free radicals, unstable molecules that damage healthy cells. Vitamin E is a powerful antioxidant that promotes healing by destroying free radicals.

Take 5,000 to 10,000 milligrams daily of vitamin C with bioflavonoids and 50,000 international units (IU) of vita-

HERBAL POWER

Soothe with Lavender

Combine the benefits of lavender (*Lavandula,* various species) essential oil and aloe vera gel to fight the pain and infection of burns, says David Winston, a founding professional member of the American Herbalists Guild and founder and president of Herbalist and Alchemist in Broadway, New Jersey. Blend one or two drops of essential oil of lavender with aloe gel scraped from a fresh plant leaf. Apply this daily to minor burns for a few days, he suggests.

Linalool and linalyl acetate, lavender's active ingredients, possess soothing and sedating qualities, adds Jeanne Rose, a San Francisco herbalist and author, executive director of the Aromatic Plant Project, and past president of the National Association for Holistic Aromatherapy. The Aromatic Plant Project encourages the growing and distillation of plants to make essential oils and plant waters, or hydrosols. For more information, write to P. O. Box 225336, San Francisco, California 94122-5336.

min A daily. Do this for about 2 weeks to promote faster healing.

Use the Bach Rescue Remedy, if you have some, or look for it in your health food store. Follow the dosage directions on the label. This multipurpose flower-essence remedy is known for its comforting and soothing effects.

Do a visualization. Imagine that the burned area is a painful, fiery red that you transform into a cool, comfortable blue.

Other Approaches

Beef up your daily calorie intake to enhance tissue healing. Eating extra helpings of carbohydrates, protein, and even fat gives your body more energy for healing burned areas, which is especially necessary if you are burned over a large part of your body, says Randolph Wong, M.D., a plastic and reconstructive surgeon and director of the burn unit at Straub Clinic and Hospital in Honolulu.

If you are soaking the burn in cool water, add some milk as well. The cool water helps get rid of the pain, and the lactic acid and sugar in the milk make the skin feel more comfortable, explains Melvin Elson, M.D., medical director of the Dermatology Center in Nashville.

Avoid putting butter or petroleum jelly on burns. While these products may feel gentle, they are risky because they spark bacteria growth that could lead to infection, warns John P. Heggers, Ph.D., professor in the department of surgery, microbiology, and immunology at the University of Texas Medical Branch and director of clinical microbiology at the Shriners Burns Institute, both in Galveston. "Butter contains salt, which draws all the water out of the cell tissues and causes them to collapse. Petroleum jelly prevents the tissue from breathing and eventually kills the tissue," he explains.

Place a ¼-inch-thick slice of raw potato directly on the minor burn area. "Raw potatoes hold in a lot of moisture and have enzymes called proteases that are used by the skin for healing," explains Mark Stengler, N.D., a naturopathic physician in Carlsbad, California, and author of *The Natural Physician*. He recommends using a fresh potato slice twice a day on the site for at least 3 days to take away redness and swelling. Keep the slice on the burn for 30 to 60 minutes, using gauze to hold it in place.

Treat erupted blisters with a mixture of 1 tablespoon of white vinegar in 1 pint of water. Ideally, you should let blisters heal by themselves, but if they do break open, this is the remedy to try, says Dr. Elson. Soak the blistered area in this mixture for 15 minutes, three or four times a day, he suggests. You can use a washcloth or compress. "This solution fights bacteria, infections, and inflammation," he says. "It should dry up the blister in a day."

Note: See a doctor if the blister fluid is white or yellow, since those colors are signs of infection.

Reach for over-the-counter antibiotic ointments such as Bacitracin or Neosporin to fight infection and swelling. Simply read the labels for directions, says Dr. Wong.

Make a garlic-and-onion paste and place it directly on the burn. These plants possess antiseptic properties, says James A. Duke, Ph.D., a botanical consultant, a former ethnobotanist with the U.S. Department of Agriculture who specializes in medicinal plants, and author of *The Green Pharmacy*. Chop up onions and garlic, then mash them with a spoon to make the paste, he advises. You can spread this paste directly on any burn from a first-degree up to a mild second-degree and leave it on for 4 hours or so. (A mild second-degree burn will appear red, swollen, and blistery, and you will feel some pain.) If the garlic causes further skin discomfort, use the onion alone, says Dr. Duke.

Drink 8 to 10 eight-ounce glasses of water daily. Your skin becomes dried out when you have a burn. The extra liquid will help prevent dehydration, says Dr. Stengler.

Once the skin heals, apply moisturizer or sunscreen daily. Over-the-counter products can help prevent scarring, according to Dr. Wong. Even the healed skin tends to be dry and fragile for the first year because burns often damage oil and sweat glands. He recommends moisturizing sunscreens that have a base of aloe.

Bursitis

Whenever you see -*itis* on the end of a word, it means "inflammation of" whatever body part begins the word. With bursitis, it is inflammation of the bursae. Bursae are fluid-filled sacs that act as buffers to prevent friction between bones, tendons, ligaments, and muscles. There are more than 150 bursae in the body, but the ones that give most folks trouble are in the shoulders, elbows, knees, and hips.

When you injure or overuse a joint, the bursae fill with even more fluid and become inflamed. The inflamed bursae put pressure on surrounding tissue, which can cause severe pain and loss of movement.

The Blended Prescription

Note: To learn about cautions and possible side effects of the remedies in this chapter, see page 253.

Bursitis generally goes away on its own in a few days or weeks—as long as you don't continue to strain the area or reinjure it. You should see your doctor if you develop a fever, severe pain, or redness in the area where you are experiencing bursitis. But even if your bursitis is not serious, you will want to feel better and do everything you can to speed up the healing process. Here is a prescription for healing and relief from our blended-medicine experts.

As soon as a bout of bursitis flares up, apply the time-tested RICE approach: Rest, Ice, Compress, Elevate.

1. Stop what you are doing and give the joint a rest. A long one. It may be hard to do, but refraining from activities that hurt is probably the fastest road to healing, says Steven Subotnick, D.P.M., N.D., Ph.D., clinical professor of biomechanics and surgery at the

HERBAL POWER

Turmeric for Pain

Some say that turmeric (*Cùrcuma longa*) is as effective as cortisone when it comes to relieving some types of inflammation. Best of all, this spice (also available in capsule form) may help protect the stomach lining from ulcer formation and against damage done by other anti-inflammatory agents, says John Collins, N.D., a naturopathic physician and a teacher of homeopathy at the National College of Naturopathic Medicine in Portland, Oregon.

You can buy the capsules in health food stores. Take 500 milligrams on an empty stomach 20 minutes before each meal until pain subsides.

California College of Podiatric Medicine in Hayward, a specialist in sports medicine, and author of *Sports and Exercise Injuries*. Don't return to an activity until you can do so without pain.

2. Ice painful areas for 20 minutes three or four times a day or until the pain and swelling go down. The cold should reduce your pain and swelling, says Dr. Subotnick. You can buy special ice packs to use on your leg; however, a plastic bag filled with ice cubes or a bag of frozen vegetables works just as well. Just make sure that you wrap whatever cold pack you use in a towel to prevent skin damage.

3. Use an elastic bandage to apply pressure to the painful joints. "The wrap will help provide heat, restrict motion, and work to 'pump out' swelling," says Dale Anderson, M.D., clinical assistant professor at the University of Minnesota Medical School in Minneapolis and author of *Muscle Pain Relief in 90 Seconds:*

SKILLFUL HEALERS

Acupuncture

Acupuncture can work wonderfully to send the pain and swelling of bursitis on its way. A practitioner might insert a needle into the body near the joint that's causing the trouble, such as the shoulder, says Kirk Moulton, a traditional Chinese medicine physician and a certified acupuncturist at American WholeHealth Centers in Chicago. You might need two or three treatments a week for the first 2 weeks. Then you may be able to scale back to about a treatment per week for another 4 weeks. Acupuncture is highly effective when combined with other efforts to heal the inflamed joint, such as rest, he says.

The Fold and Hold Method. To make sure that the bandage isn't on too tight, check your circulation every 15 minutes or so by squeezing your big toe or one of the fingers on the bandaged leg or arm. Make sure that it returns to its normal color when you release it. If it remains white, loosen the bandage immediately.

4. Keep the injured area elevated for the first 24 to 48 hours. Propping your leg or arm on two pillows or a soft chair will minimize swelling, says Dr. Subotnick. Even while in bed, prop your injured area up with a bunch of pillows.

To relieve pain, take the homeopathic remedy Arnica 6C. Take two pellets every 15 minutes until pain improves, then two pellets every 4 hours until the bursitis subsides.

To reduce swelling, tenderness, and pain, apply arnica (*Arnica montana*) ointment or Traumed ointment to the affected area four or five times a day. Both are available in health food stores.

Curb the pain with an over-the-counter painkiller.
Our experts recommend two 200-milligram tablets of
ibuprofen every 4 hours until the pain goes away. Then
continue taking your painkiller for no more than 10 days
at a time, closer to 6-hour intervals. Most people quit
taking the medicine as soon as the pain starts to go away,
Dr. Anderson says, but that can lead to a recurrence.

**To reduce inflammation, take bromelain, an enzyme
available in supplement form that is known to improve circulation and treat inflammation.** Take two 375-milligram
capsules at a potency of 2,400 mcu (a standard unit of
measurement for enzymes) three times a day between
meals as long as needed. Bromelain takes a few days to
start working, but once it does, it is one of the most effective agents available for reducing pain and inflammation.

Pour in some ginger. Ginger (*Zingiber officinale*) extract
is another natural anti-inflammatory supplement you may
want to try. Take one 250-milligram capsule twice a day.
It works particularly well in conjunction with bromelain.

Other Approaches

**Use the Fold and Hold method for 90 seconds, three
times a day, until your pain is gone.** The Fold and Hold
method helps relax and relieve tension from the muscles
surrounding the area where you have bursitis, says Dr. Anderson. To perform it, follow these directions (the expla-
nations in parentheses explain the process for the
shoulder, but you can use this for any joint).

- Find the tender spot. (This could be difficult to find
  in the shoulder because there are a bunch of bones
  under which the tender spot could hide. Or it could
  be in the deep, thick muscles along the back of the
  shoulder.)

- Put yourself in a position that makes the tender spot feel better. (For shoulder bursitis, raising your arm above your head is often the most comfortable position. It might hurt to get it there if you lift it out from the side, so try lifting it out in front of you as you raise it. Most people benefit by pointing the thumb of their raised arm toward their back.)
- Hold that position for at least 90 seconds. (For the shoulder, lie down or lean against a wall on the raised-arm side of your body. This pushes the shoulder further toward the center of the body, says Dr. Anderson.)
- Gently and slowly return to a normal position.

Take 2,000 to 3,000 milligrams of vitamin C two or three times a day. Vitamin C in large doses helps with structural healing, says John Collins, N.D., a naturopathic physician and a teacher of homeopathy at the National College of Naturopathic Medicine in Portland, Oregon. Take this dose of vitamin C for the first week or two of your bursitis.

Take 1,000 milligrams of mixed bioflavonoids for as long as you have inflammation plus a few days afterward. Bioflavonoids include such things as grapeseed extract and pine bark extract. "These are perfectly safe to take long-term," says Dr. Collins. They work well with vitamin C to reduce swelling and pain, he says. Bioflavonoids take a few days to start working, but if you keep taking them, you should see marked improvement. You can buy them in most health food stores.

Canker Sores

Stress, hormonal fluctuations, and lowered immunity have often been blamed for causing canker sores, but no one is really sure what makes them take up housekeeping in the warm, moist interior of the mouth. These tiny ulcerations—also called aphthous ulcers—usually occur between cheek and gum. The small, swollen red sores often hang around for 10 to 14 days. While they don't cause other health complications, they can be acutely painful.

The Blended Prescription

Note: To learn about cautions and possible side effects of the remedies in this chapter, see page 253.

If a sore is not healed within 14 days or is accompanied by fever, nausea, or swollen neck glands, see your physician or dentist. Meanwhile, you can take some action to ease the pain. Here's a five-step approach from our blended-medicine experts that taps the best of prescription medications, herbs, and plain common sense.

Rinse your mouth with warm, slightly salted water. Salt seems to have an anti-inflammatory effect on canker sores, says Meena Shah, D.D.S., a dentist in Lake Grove, New York. Mix about ½ teaspoon of salt in one glass of moderately warm water. Stir to dissolve the salt, then gently swish a mouthful. Repeat three to five times daily until the sore is healed, Dr. Shah advises.

Apply one drop of tea tree (*Melaleuca alternifolia*) oil directly to the sore to help guard against further infection. Be careful here: This is a strong essential oil, so use no more than one drop and let it sit on the sore and dissipate in your mouth, as opposed to quickly swallowing.

Avoid acid-forming foods such as citrus, sugar, alcohol, and chewing gum.

For an herbal remedy, take 200 milligrams of echinacea (*Echinacea*, various species) three times a day. This herb helps to boost immunity.

If you want to escalate the battle, ask your doctor about amlexanox (Aphthasol), a new prescription paste. It can be applied several times a day.

Colds

There are roughly 200 cold viruses, each with a slightly different effect on your body. But your body's response to them doesn't vary much, which is why they are all lumped together under one name: the common cold. Cold viruses enter your body via the air (someone has coughed or sneezed nearby) or your fingers (you touched a surface where a cold virus was sitting and then touched your eyes, nose, or mouth). Once in your body, the virus latches on to mucous membranes that line your nose and throat and quickly multiply.

The discomfort of colds is not from the virus itself but from your body's response to the infection. White blood cells quickly fire off chemical weapons called histamines to kill the fast-growing virus colony. It is the histamines that cause nasal and sinus inflammation, chest congestion, sore throat, and fatigue.

The Blended Prescription

Note: To learn about cautions and possible side effects of the remedies in this chapter, see page 253.

If you have a high fever, your illness is not just a cold. If you can't swallow or eat or breathe, it is not just a cold.

And if it hurts really badly in your head or chest, it is not just a cold. In such cases, see a doctor.

Usually, you know when it is a cold. To fight it, you need to relieve the symptoms induced by histamines and stimulate your immune system to fight the infection. Here is a six-step core program from our panel of blended-medicine experts to make a cold go away fast.

Give yourself 48 hours—consecutive hours—for rest, relaxation, and healing. The stresses of work and activity diminish your immune system. By calming down your life for 2 days, you give your body the time and energy to heal itself. And by sequestering yourself, you do the world a favor by not spreading your germs.

Sip liquids constantly throughout your waking hours. Hot liquids like herbal tea and chicken soup are best for several reasons: They diminish a virus's ability to replicate, they soothe the throat, and the warmth helps decongest the nasal passages and lungs. Water is beneficial as well.

Help yourself to 1,000 milligrams of vitamin C every 2 to 4 hours. You can start this dose at the first sign of sniffles. And if you continue for 3 to 4 days after you feel better, you will help prevent a relapse.

Vitamin C jump-starts the immune system by arming white blood cells with the right ammunition to fend off colds and other infections. And it is an antihistamine that helps dry up watery eyes and a runny nose.

Take high dosages of the herb echinacea (*Echinacea purpurea*). Studies have shown that this herb helps improve the body's immune system so that it is better able to ward off attackers like cold viruses. (For details, see "Herbal Power" on page 56.)

Take one or two 15-milligram zinc gluconate lozenges (such as Cold-Eeze) at the first sign of discomfort, then take them every 2 hours until you feel better. If your head is pounding, your throat is sore, and your nose is stuffy, continue this treatment throughout your waking hours for 1 week. Be sure to suck on the lozenges until they are completely dissolved in your mouth, or they won't be as effective.

In one study, participants who sucked on one zinc gluconate lozenge (containing 13.3 milligrams of zinc) every 2 hours while awake throughout their colds got rid of their coughs, nasal congestion, sore throats, and headaches 3 to 4 days sooner than those in the placebo group.

HERBAL POWER

Fight with Echinacea

Also referred to as the purple coneflower plant, echinacea (*Echinacea purpurea*) is a potent herb that should take center stage in your line of defense against the cold. Studies have shown that this centuries-old herb is a powerhouse when it comes to bolstering immunity. "Echinacea stimulates the production of white blood cells to kill viruses," says David Field, N.D., a naturopathic physician and licensed acupuncturist in Santa Rosa, California.

The moment you feel sneezy and stuffy, "take two 200-milligram capsules of echinacea every 2 hours for the first 24 hours. On the second day, take the same dosage every 4 hours, and then every 6 hours after that while cold symptoms last," suggests Michael Traub, N.D., a naturopathic physician in Kailua Kona, Hawaii.

You can also use echinacea in tincture form. Place 40 drops in a 6- to 8-ounce glass of water or juice. Repeat the dose every 2 hours. On the second day, drink the mixture every 4 hours and every 6 hours thereafter, Dr. Traub says.

Inhale the steam from eucalyptus (*Eucalyptus globulus*) essential oil and water. The key to eucalyptus's healing power is a chemical called cineole, or eucalyptol, which aids in the loosening of mucus. Put 10 to 15 drops of eucalyptus oil in a pan of water, heat to boiling, and remove the pan from the stove. Covering your head with a towel and leaning over the pan, inhale the steam through your nostrils—and blow your nose frequently. Repeat the steam inhalation three or four times daily. Be careful not to let the steam burn your face or sinuses while taking this steam bath.

Other Approaches

Take 200,000 international units (IU) of beta-carotene at the beginning stages of a cold. "It strengthens immunity and probably has some antiviral effects as well," says David Edelberg, M.D., assistant professor of medicine at Rush Medical College in Chicago and chairman and founder of the American WholeHealth Centers in Chicago, Boston, Denver, and Bethesda, Maryland.

Beta-carotene can also help prevent secondary infections associated with colds. After the first large dose, take 25,000 IU daily until symptoms resolve, suggests Michael Traub, N.D., a naturopathic physician in Kailua Kona, Hawaii.

Use cough suppressants, mild decongestants, or over-the-counter remedies such as acetaminophen as needed for headache and sinus pain. "Most over-the-counter remedies relieve symptoms," says Dr. Traub. That includes multisymptom cold medicines, which often provide relief just as advertised. But those drugstore remedies won't work with the body to heal itself, and colds could last longer when these medications are used, he cautions. For fast healing, look at some of the alternatives.

SKILLFUL HEALERS

Acupuncture

Acupuncture can be just what you need to relieve nasty cold symptoms, says David Field, N.D., a naturopathic physician and licensed acupuncturist in Santa Rosa, California. "It can put an end to nasal congestion and inflamed mucous membranes, coughing, and fatigue."

To tackle congestion, the acupuncturist may insert needles into your sinus area along both sides of your nose, says David Molony, Ph.D., executive director of the American Association of Oriental Medicine and a licensed acupuncturist in Catasauqua, Pennsylvania. Or he may apply needles to the acupuncture point between your eyebrows.

To suppress a hacking cough, the acupuncturist may even insert needles on certain points along your wrist. "In about 24 to 48 hours, your cold symptoms should be gone," Dr. Molony says.

As soon as cold symptoms strike, take 300 milligrams of garlic powder in capsule or tablet form three times a day until the symptoms have disappeared completely. Studies show that this herb can prevent and even stamp out a cold in its earliest stages, says Dr. Traub. Garlic powder yields allicin, one of nature's strongest antibiotics, and it has several compounds that help mobilize white blood cells.

If you are buying garlic supplements, make sure that the capsules or tablets have an enteric coating, a protective shell that allows the supplement to dissolve more slowly in your digestive tract. You get the most therapeutic effects that way, explains Dr. Traub.

To get more potent benefits, eat two to three raw garlic

cloves per meal for 1 to 2 days, suggests David Field, N.D., a naturopathic physician and licensed acupuncturist in Santa Rosa, California. Mince the raw cloves and sprinkle them over pasta or soups.

Three times daily, take one 250- to 500-milligram capsule of 10 percent alkaloid goldenseal (*Hydrastis canadensis*). You should begin taking this dose at the first sign of cold symptoms and continue until your symptoms clear up, says William D. Nelson, N.D., a naturopathic physician in Colorado Springs, Colorado. Or mix 1 to 1½ teaspoons of the tincture in 8 ounces of water three times a day, he suggests.

One of nature's more bitter herbs, goldenseal contains antibacterial and antibiotic-like compounds. It is known for stimulating white blood cell production. It can help dry up nasal and sinus secretions and reduce the swelling of mucous membranes, says Liz Collins, N.D., a naturopathic physician and co-owner of the Natural Childbirth and Family Clinic in Portland, Oregon.

Try the homeopathic remedy Oscillococcinum. It's a pill you can take twice a day for 3 days, says Earl Mindell, Ph.D., professor of nutrition at Pacific Western University in Los Angeles and author of *Earl Mindell's Supplement Bible*. Available in some drugstores and health food stores, this remedy eliminates many cold symptoms and helps you get over your cold more quickly. "Place these tiny pills under your tongue, where they dissolve very rapidly," he suggests. "Before you know it, your body begins producing antibodies to fight the cold."

Add 20 drops each of eucalyptus (*Eucalyptus globulus*), lavender (*Lavandula officinalis*), and clary sage (*Salvia sclarea*) essential oils to your bathwater. This aromatherapy mixture can help you feel better by melting away the fatigue associated with cold symptoms, according to Michael Scholes, president of the Michael Scholes

School of Aromatic Studies in Los Angeles. For a totally relaxing and aromatic experience, fill a tub with your favorite bubble bath, pour in the mixture of essential oils, and soak in the bath for 20 minutes or so. The combination will strengthen your immune system and strip away fatigue, he says.

Gently massage the area around your nose. This acupressure technique will help relieve congestion, says David Molony, Ph.D., executive director of the American Association of Oriental Medicine and a licensed acupuncturist in Catasauqua, Pennsylvania. After you have massaged your nose area for about 5 minutes, move your fingers up to your scalp. Beginning 1 inch above your hairline, lightly massage your scalp for another 5 minutes. You can repeat these steps as often as you like to get relief, he says.

You can also relieve congestion by massaging the webbed area between your thumb and index finger for 5 minutes, Dr. Molony says.

Use either of these techniques as often as you like and for as long as you have cold symptoms. The effects of acupressure can last for a couple of hours, especially if you perform them right before bedtime, Dr. Molony says. You will encourage a good night's sleep, which is an essential part of getting yourself well.

Cold Sores

Cold sores actually start inside the body with exposure to or activation of the contagious virus called herpes simplex type 1. When an outbreak is about to arrive, you will sense an ominous tingling in the doomed site. Within days, a blistery sore erupts, often outside the mouth at the margins of the lips. Unsightly and painful, cold sores run their course in a week or more.

The Blended Prescription

Note: To learn about cautions and possible side effects of the remedies in this chapter, see page 253.

As the pain prods away at your lip, you can take immediate action to ease your discomfort as well as use tactics that will keep the cold sores from coming back. Here is a three-part prescription from our blended-medicine experts.

Apply lemon balm (*Melissa officinalis*) ointment several times during the day. Or dab the sore once or twice a day with a cotton swab dipped in a petroleum jelly like Vaseline. Both promote healing and soothe cracked skin.

At the first sign of a cold sore inside your mouth, suck on a 15-milligram zinc gluconate lozenge (such as Cold-Eeze) until it dissolves. Then repeat every 3 to 4 hours as needed until the symptoms are gone. Zinc boosts immunity. Since colds sores are caused by a virus, higher immunity may help fight them off.

Have an herbal supplement of 200 milligrams of echinacea (*Echinacea*, various species) three times a day. This will help your immune system battle against the herpes virus.

Constipation

For food to be properly digested, it needs to encounter a number of chemicals as it works its way toward the colon. Among them are beneficial bacteria, stomach acid, pancreatic enzymes, and the yellowish substance called bile, which comes from the liver. If these partners have done their work, food wastes are almost in the form of a stool by the time they reach your colon. There, your colon muscles quickly contract to move the waste to your rectum, which signals the brain that you need to get to a bathroom. But sometimes this digestive trip gets off track, and your colon holds on to waste.

When those stools remain in the colon for more than a few hours, they start to dehydrate and harden from lack of fluids. Occasionally, they develop rough edges that can cause microscopic tears in your rectum. That explains why bowel movements can be painful for someone who has

---

HERBAL POWER

The Roots of Relief

Rely on the triple talents of dandelion (*Taraxacum officinale*), gentian (*Gentiana*, various species), and ginger (*Zingiber officinale*) to restore normal digestion. These three roots, taken together or separately, motivate the stomach to produce acid, the pancreas to produce enzymes, and the liver to produce bile—all key digestive steps, says Mark Stengler, N.D., a naturopathic physician in Carlsbad, California, and author of *The Natural Physician*.

For best results for chronic constipation, take one 250-milligram capsule each of dandelion, gentian, and ginger with meals until the constipation is corrected, says Dr. Stengler. If you prefer taking them in tincture form, try 30 drops of each. These herbs address long-term constipation by improving digestion and the spontaneous movement of the intestine (motility).

been constipated: When you flex the muscles to move your bowels, the hard stools start scraping away at tender internal tissues.

The Blended Prescription

Note: To learn about cautions and possible side effects of the remedies in this chapter, see page 253.

Constipation usually can be self-treated. See your doctor if there is any mucus, blood, or undigested food in the stool; if the stool itself is consistently pencil thin (this could be a sign of colon cancer or a blockage); or if you have not passed a stool for more than 3 days past your normal defecation cycle.

So how can you get things moving on your own? There are really two sets of prescriptions. One is for the person who is dealing with a one-time case of constipation brought on by traveling, increased stress, or a change in diet. If that describes you, try the following four tips from our blended-medicine experts to get the stool out of your system.

Take ½ teaspoon of the herb cascara sagrada (*Rhamnus purshianus*) at bedtime. But don't use it regularly, as your colon may become dependent on it. Cascara sagrada is a popular, time-tested laxative herb used in dozens of over-the-counter constipation remedies.

Pick up Citrate of Magnesia or Fleet Phospha-soda at the drugstore and follow the package instructions. These laxatives work by drawing water into the intestines, causing increased pressure and stimulation, which gets things moving.

For a homeopathic solution, try Calcarea carb. 6C. Take two pellets every 15 minutes for four doses, then two pellets every hour for the rest of the day. After that, take two pellets four times a day until symptoms subside. Use for no more than 5 days.

If after a few days (4 or 5, depending on your comfort level) you experience no relief, give yourself a Fleet enema, following the instructions on the package. Don't use this method repeatedly, however.

If you find that constipation is ongoing rather than sporadic, try the following blend, which works best for chronic constipation.

Twice a day, take 1 tablespoon of a psyllium-husk product (such as Metamucil). Psyllium is a type of fiber that softens and bulks up stools for easier passing.

Drink 6 to 12 ounces of prune juice daily, or regularly eat prunes and figs. These two fruits provide fiber and help keep everything moving.

Take 3,000 to 4,000 milligrams of vitamin C daily. At high doses, vitamin C creates loose stools. If this causes diarrhea for more than 3 days, see a doctor.

Consciously increase the fiber in your diet. Eat more raw fruits, grains, and raw vegetables.

Drink plenty of water—ideally, eight 8-ounce glasses every day.

Other Approaches

Eat two apples and one banana a day. These fiber-packed fruits are high in pectin, a slippery substance that helps stools slide out of your bowels, explains David Molony, Ph.D., executive director of the American Association of Oriental Medicine and a licensed acupuncturist in Catasauqua, Pennsylvania. Eat this amount of fruit until you can move your bowels easily, he advises. If you are prone to constipation, make these foods a consistent part of your diet.

Have a flaxseed-and-oatmeal breakfast. Add 1 teaspoon of ground flaxseed to 1 quart of water, bring it to a boil, and simmer for 15 minutes. Then add rolled oats to the water, following the directions on the box, and continue cooking until the oatmeal is cooked. This makes about 2 cups of oatmeal. If you want a smaller serving, use less water. This healthy breakfast soothes irritated intestines and may help unblock bowel movements, says Dr. Molony.

Drink three large glasses of warm or room-temperature water in half an hour. The rapid water consumption helps to stimulate a bowel movement, says Dr. Molony.

Put 10 to 15 drops of Angostura bitters in 2 ounces of juice or water, and drink this mixture before every meal. The gentian (an herb) in the bitters works best to stimulate bile secretion and bowel movement for people with chronic constipation, says David Winston, a founding professional member of the American Herbalists Guild and founder and president of Herbalist and Alchemist in Broadway, New Jersey. "Bitters must be tasted—not taken in capsule form—to work best," he adds. Angostura bitters can be purchased at grocery and liquor stores.

Take two capsules of garlic (300 to 400 milligrams per capsule) twice a day with your largest meals. Garlic works to kill harmful bacteria in the colon, says Jennifer Brett, N.D., a naturopathic physician in Norwalk and Stratford, Connecticut. Some bacteria can cause changes in stool consistency. Others release toxic by-products that can cause cramping of the large intestine. Garlic also increases bile flow into the intestines. Bile is a natural stool softener, and increasing the flow speeds up the rate of elimination of the bowel contents, she explains.

Do up to 50 abdominal crunches daily. Toned abdominal muscles assist the digestive system in passing stools, says Mark Stengler, N.D., a naturopathic physician in

Carlsbad, California, and author of *The Natural Physician*. Lie on top of a bench with your knees over one end and your feet planted on the floor (or lie on the floor with your knees bent and your feet on the floor). Resting your hands lightly on your abdomen, lift your shoulders slowly and slightly, then hold for a few seconds. At the tips of your fingers, you should feel the abdominal muscles contract. Continue doing the crunches until you feel a burn in your abdomen. Then relax for 30 seconds and resume. Try to work up to 25, repeated twice a day, Dr. Stengler recommends. Do not pull your head up with your hands—this could cause neck injury, he cautions.

Eat a sprig of fennel with dinner. In some fine restaurants, a sprig of fennel is used as a garnish on plates of pasta. This herb, which grows wild in some parts of California, stimulates secretions to enhance bowel movements, says Dr. Molony. "It can really get things moving inside you." Check your produce aisle for this garnish, and have a sprig with your meal. It is also good as a breath freshener after a meal, he adds.

Cuts, Scrapes, and Scratches

As protective as your skin is, it is no match for a slip of a kitchen carving knife, cat scratches, or a tumble on a gravel driveway. When your top layer of skin, the epidermis, gets sliced or scraped, your body sounds an alarm answered immediately by your white blood cells. Like ambulance paramedics, the white blood cells—along with red blood cells and platelets—rush to the wound site to help form a clot and start the healing process. The dam-

HERBAL POWER

Clean with Calendula

The bright yellow- and orange-flowered calendula, also known as pot marigold, is an effective herb for treating cuts, scrapes, and scratches, says Mark Stengler, N.D., a naturopathic physician in Carlsbad, California, and author of *The Natural Physician*.

After cleaning the wound with soap and water, put several drops of a nonalcohol-based calendula (*Calendula officinalis*) tincture on the wound two or three times a day, Dr. Stengler prescribes. "Calendula is a natural antiseptic," he notes. This herb also motivates the immune system to increase the supply of white blood cells. The tincture version of calendula works especially well on wide cuts, he says.

aged epidermis sloughs off while healthy skin edges into an area now covered by a protective scab. Toiling day and night, your cells multiply, laying down a meshwork of tissue that eventually fills the gap and becomes covered by new, protective skin.

The Blended Prescription

Note: To learn about cautions and possible side effects of the remedies in this chapter, see page 253.

When you have an open wound, your first objective is to stop the bleeding. If the cut is deep, place a clean towel or sterile bandage on top of the wound and hold it firmly. Bleeding should stop in 5 to 10 minutes.

If the bleeding is hard to control or you have a cut that is long, wide, and nasty-looking, maintain the pressure on the wound and get to an emergency room. A deep cut might need some stitches, and the suturing must be done promptly. Highly contaminated wounds may not bleed but are potentially dangerous.

For minor, run-of-the-mill cuts, scrapes, and scratches, however, try this powerful five-step healing program from our blended-medicine experts.

Fill a small bowl with a cup of cool water, and clean the wound with a clean washcloth or sterile gauze or cotton. If it's available, add 10 drops of tea tree (*Melaleuca alternifolia*) essential oil to the water before cleansing the wound. Its antiseptic properties are similar to hydrogen peroxide.

After cleaning, apply an over-the-counter antibiotic ointment like Bacitracin. Other good choices to discourage infection are calendula (*Calendula officinalis*) cream and aloe vera gel.

Cover lightly with a bandage.

Take 1,000 milligrams of vitamin C three times a day. This supplement bolsters your body's immune system.

To help speed healing, supplement with 400 international units (IU) of vitamin E. Take this vitamin twice a day until the wound heals.

Other Approaches

Cover the wound initially, then treat it with a sugar-Betadine mixture to discourage scarring. After you have cleaned the wound, cover it with gauze. Wait 12 to 24 hours to ensure that no bleeding is present, then gently clean the wound again. Now you are ready for the healing mix.

In a double boiler, gently warm 1 tablespoon of Betadine solution and 3 tablespoons of Betadine ointment, then add 10 tablespoons of white granular table sugar as the mixture cools, says Richard A. Knutson, M.D., an orthopedic surgeon at Delta Medical Center in Greenville,

Mississippi. Apply the cooled mixture two to four times a day as needed, he suggests. Sugar takes away water from bacteria, which hastens their death, and strips bacteria of the necessary nutrients that they need to multiply. Store the ointment at room temperature in a covered container.

Treat scrapes with hydrogen peroxide. If your knee meets the pavement, scraping that protective top layer of skin off your knee, blood and yellowish-to-clear fluids may ooze from the wound. To keep the wound clean and give it the best chance of healing well, pour on a capful of hydrogen peroxide or dab the site with cotton swabs soaked in this solution. Follow up by washing with soap and water.

"Hydrogen peroxide is a good cleaning agent that bubbles out debris," says John McCabe, M.D., professor of emergency medicine at the State University of New York Health Science Center at Syracuse. "By cleaning the scrape, you help lay down a good foundation for growing new skin with less scarring."

Eat protein daily to help heal cuts, scrapes, and scratches. Adequate amounts of protein in your diet are important because protein contains amino acids that help build skin and tissue in the wound area, says Mark Michaud, M.D., a family physician with American WholeHealth Centers in Chicago. Good sources of low-fat protein include whole-grain millet, fish, beans, nuts, tofu, and grains.

If you generally eat 50 grams of protein a day, raise the amount to 100 grams a day until you heal properly, advises Michele Gottschlich, R.D., Ph.D., director of nutrition services for the Shriners Burns Institute in Cincinnati.

Dandruff

On your scalp, skin cells grow, multiply, and die each day. Usually, the dead cells flake away invisibly as living cells emerge to the skin's surface. But when cells grow and die off too rapidly, visible dandruff appears in the form of tiny white flakes of skin that fall onto your collar and shoulders.

The Blended Prescription

Note: To learn about cautions and possible side effects of the remedies in this chapter, see page 253.

Despite the embarrassment, dandruff is harmless. Stress, food allergies, yeast infections, and heredity are some of the most common triggers. Overactive oil glands in the scalp and high levels of the fungus *Pityrosporum ovale* are linked to the more severe cases. See your doctor if your flakes are itchy, thick, greasy, and yellow. Those are signs of seborrheic dermatitis, an inflammatory scalp condition. Also see your doctor if you have dry, thick lesions that itch like crazy and leave your scalp red and inflamed. Those are symptoms of psoriasis, a recurrent skin disease.

If all you have is an average case of dandruff, though, here is a surefire four-step prescription from our blended-medicine experts to get those flakes under control, now and forever.

For a fast solution, use an antidandruff shampoo. Choose one that contains coal tar, salicylic acid, pyrithione zinc, selenium sulfide, or sulfur, says Patricia Farris Walters, M.D., clinical assistant professor of dermatology at Tulane University School of Medicine in New Orleans.

The tar-based shampoos slow down cell production, while salicylic acid–based shampoos slough off dead cells

HERBAL POWER

Brew a Hair Tonic

In a nonaluminum pot, boil 4 heaping tablespoons of dried thyme (*Thymus vulgaris*) in 2 cups of water for 10 minutes. Strain it and allow the tea to cool. Pour the brew over damp, freshly shampooed hair and gently massage it into your scalp. You don't need to rinse. Thyme is an herb that is very effective at controlling dandruff, says Chris Meletis, N.D., professor of natural pharmacology and nutrition, dean of clinical education, and chief medical officer at the National College of Naturopathic Medicine in Portland, Oregon. You can also use 2 tablespoons of fresh rosemary or sage instead of thyme.

before they clump. Both shampoos have antifungal properties to help fight yeast, which is one of dandruff's most persistent triggers. Pyrithione zinc and selenium sulfide reduce cell turnover, while sulfur is believed to cause slight skin irritation—just enough to lead to the shedding of flakes.

For a long-term solution, take 1 tablespoon daily of either flaxseed (*Linum usitatissimum*) oil, evening primrose (*Oenothera biennis*) oil, borage (*Borago officinalis*) oil, or omega-3 fish oil. Or take nine 1,000-milligram capsules of one of these oils each day, says Chris Meletis, N.D., professor of natural pharmacology and nutrition, dean of clinical education, and chief medical officer at the National College of Naturopathic Medicine in Portland, Oregon. These oils, called essential fatty acids, can prevent the rapid shedding of dead skin cells by promoting the growth of healthier skin tissues from the outset, he says. Understand, though, that this solution might take up to 3 months to take effect. If there is little or no change after 3 months, switch to a different oil.

Swallow 1 to 2 milligrams of biotin a day. Biotin maintains healthy skin and can control dandruff buildup by improving the metabolism of scalp oils, which play a role in manufacturing those itchy white flakes, says Dr. Meletis.

In addition, consider washing your hair with biotin shampoo. Dandruff may be a sign of a biotin deficiency, says Michael Traub, N.D., a naturopathic physician in Kailua Kona, Hawaii. As with the essential fatty acids, biotin supplements could take up to 3 months before having an effect.

Make sure that you are getting the following vitamins and minerals. They will provide the nutritional support you need for healthy skin and can help foster correction of dandruff.

Vitamin A: 5,000 international units (IU) per day

Vitamin E: 400 IU per day

Zinc: 30 to 50 milligrams per day

Other Approaches

Conduct a diet test to see if a food allergy is causing the problem. "Food allergies often manifest themselves as skin ailments, including dandruff," says Dr. Meletis. Some foods prompt the immune system to release histamines, which cause skin inflammation and itching. So if you clean up your diet, you remove the cause and can get your dandruff under control, he says.

How to proceed? Eliminate all dairy products, eggs, peanuts, and wheat from your diet for 10 to 21 days. If your dandruff goes away, reintroduce the foods one at a time, 3 days apart. If a reintroduced food aggravates your dandruff, eliminate that food for an additional 3 months and then reintroduce it. Most foods that can prompt a dandruff-causing reaction when eaten regularly will not flare things up after a long elimination period.

Diarrhea

Each person has a unique bathroom schedule: Some adults need to defecate three times a day; others, just a few times a week. Diarrhea is defined as stools that are more fluid or more frequent than what is usual for a person.

Any number of things can cause diarrhea, but intestinal infections, bacteria in food or drink, medications, and food allergies (particularly to dairy products) are among the most common triggers. These agents throw the intestines' program of secretion and absorption into disarray. The result is that food and liquid pass too quickly through the digestive system, causing loose, watery stools and frequent trips to the bathroom.

Diarrhea is good in that it helps rid the body of germs or chemicals that don't belong there. It is troublesome in that it dehydrates the body as well as drains it of important minerals such as potassium, sodium, magnesium, and calcium.

The Blended Prescription

Note: To learn about cautions and possible side effects of the remedies in this chapter, see page 253.

You can tame most episodes of diarrhea using this three-step sequence from our blended-medicine experts. But see a doctor if your symptoms last more than 3 days or include any of the following: fever over 101°F; severe cramps or vomiting; blood, pus, or mucus in your stool; or signs of dehydration (like cracked lips or constant, extreme thirst). Also check with your doctor if you have recently changed medications, since some drugs may cause diarrhea.

Take 1 to 2 teaspoons of Pepto-Bismol every hour until you have taken up to five doses. This over-the-counter stomach soother will help ease diarrhea symptoms. (And don't worry if your stool turns black; this is normal.) Or try Imodium, another over-the-counter antidiarrheal, following the dosage instructions on the package.

Take 1 tablespoon of a psyllium-husk product (like Metamucil) twice a day with plenty of fluids. Fiber is necessary for well-formed, easy-to-pass stools.

Try the homeopathic remedy Phosphoric acid 6C. Take two pellets every hour for four doses on the first day. After that, take two pellets three times a day until symptoms subside.

HERBAL POWER

Elm and Marshmallow

Combine the soothing herbal powers of slippery elm (*Ulmus rubra*) and marshmallow root (*Althaea officinalis*), recommends Mark Stengler, N.D., a naturopathic physician in Carlsbad, California, and author of *The Natural Physician*.

This herbal tandem heals the digestive tract lining, he says. For best results, take two 250-milligram capsules or 60 drops of tincture (in a quarter glass of warm water) of each herb four times a day until the diarrhea subsides.

Other Approaches

Drink liquids like Gatorade or Recharge to replace your lost fluids, electrolytes, and glucose. An acute case of diarrhea can quickly dehydrate you and rob your body of potassium and sodium, says Mark Stengler, N.D., a naturopathic physician in Carlsbad, California, and author of *The Natural Physician*.

Stick with the BRAT diet for diarrhea flare-ups. BRAT stands for bananas, rice, applesauce, and toast. These foods tend to be constipating and are ideal to eat when you have diarrhea, says Dr. Stengler. Start with small to moderate portions, he adds.

Drink rice water for minor diarrhea. "Rice water is a good source of minerals, including potassium," says Jennifer Brett, N.D., a naturopathic physician in Norwalk and Stratford, Connecticut. Rice helps the stool have a normal consistency and helps provide needed B vitamins, she adds.

To make rice water: Boil ½ cup of brown rice in 3 cups of water for 45 minutes. Strain out the rice and let the liquid cool. (You should have about 1 cup of rice water.) Drink 3 cups of this rice water during the day. To make a full day's supply, triple the recipe, says Dr. Brett. You may eat the rice if you choose (see BRAT diet above), but it is the rice water that does the trick.

Eat a bowl of applesauce sprinkled with nutmeg. "Nutmeg tends to put the parasites in diarrhea to sleep," says David Molony, Ph.D., executive director of the American Association of Oriental Medicine and a licensed acupuncturist in Catasauqua, Pennsylvania. This spice helps dry intestinal secretions and suppress the muscular contractions that cause bowel movements, and the applesauce contains soothing pectin.

Take Podophyllum 12X or 30C during the early stages of diarrhea. This homeopathic treatment is best used for painless, watery stools that do not leave you feeling nauseated, says Jennifer Jacobs, M.D., a homeopathic physician, assistant clinical professor of epidemiology at the University of Washington in Edmonds, and coauthor of *Healing with Homeopathy*. Take one dose of either potency after each unformed stool. You should start to feel better within 8 hours, she says.

Take 1 teaspoon of acidophilus powder in water twice a day on an empty stomach. This supplement replaces the good bacteria in your body that get overrun by the invasion of bad bacteria in your colon, says Jill Stansbury, N.D., a naturopathic physician in Battle Ground, Washington, and assistant professor and chairman of the botanical medicine department at the National College of Naturopathic Medicine in Portland, Oregon.

Take two 250-milligram capsules of activated charcoal every 2 hours for acute diarrhea that you think is the result of food poisoning. Charcoal capsules help to remove toxins in the colon and bloodstream caused by the bacterial infection, says Dr. Stengler. The capsules will cause black stools. Do not take them for longer than 7 days, he cautions.

Four times a day, take two 250-milligram capsules of goldenseal (*Hydrastis canadensis*) or 60 drops of its tincture in a quarter glass of warm water. This herb contains a chemical called berberine that fights bacteria and viruses, says Dr. Stengler. It also stimulates your immune system. If you are sensitive to the alcohol base of the tincture, let the mixture stand for 3 minutes, which allows some of the alcohol to evaporate.

Lie flat on your back or in a comfortable reclining chair and place a hot-water bottle on your abdomen for 20 minutes. "The hot water gets enzymes moving and speeds up

SKILLFUL HEALERS

Acupuncture

"The reason some people have diarrhea is that their bodies are not in balance," says David Molony, Ph.D., executive director of the American Association of Oriental Medicine and a licensed acupuncturist in Catasauqua, Pennsylvania. According to Dr. Molony, many chronic cases of diarrhea can be corrected by acupuncture and Chinese herbs. "We work to bring a sense of balance in the body and a return to normal," he says.

If you are being treated for diarrhea, an acupuncturist will insert needles into your abdominal area. You will feel only a mild skin sensation like a mosquito bite, if anything at all, says Dr. Molony. Some treatments last as long as 45 minutes, though the time will depend on your specific symptoms.

the digestive process," says Dr. Molony. "This will help food digest properly instead of running right through you." For the best effect, use very hot tap water in the hot-water bottle. Protect your abdomen with a towel, and place another towel on top of the hot-water bottle to help keep in the heat.

Alternate between a hot shower and a cold, damp towel. "If you got your diarrhea from a bad bug, you may kill the infection faster with hydrotherapy because it increases the circulation of blood, lymph, and immune cells," says Dr. Stengler. Begin with the hot treatment first—taking a comfortably hot shower for 5 minutes. Get out and quickly dry yourself. Wet a towel with cold water, wring it out, and wrap it around your midsection from your armpits to your groin. Finally, to avoid getting chilled, cover yourself with a wool blanket and keep it on for about 20 minutes, or until the towel feels warm.

Diverticular Disease

When dry, rough stools make their way through the colon, they can create weak spots in the colon wall. Over time, these weak spots can evolve into pea-size pouches known as diverticula. Chances are that you don't know you have diverticulosis (meaning you have these small pouches in your colon). It is generally symptomless. But if the pouches become inflamed or infected, it means that you have diverticulitis, a more serious condition. Diverticulitis is marked by abdominal pain as well as vomiting, fever, nausea, chills, constipation or diarrhea, and possibly blood in your stool. Severe diverticulitis may require hospitalization and even surgery.

The Blended Prescription

Note: To learn about cautions and possible side effects of the remedies in this chapter, see page 253.

If you have the symptoms above, your doctor can run tests to determine the severity of the problem. While a bad case of diverticulitis requires close care from a doctor, people with diverticula can do much on their own to avoid painful infections and to rebuild the colon walls. For those with diverticula, here is a six-part prescription from our panel of blended-medicine experts.

Eat a high-fiber diet, totaling 25 to 40 grams of fiber a day. Most doctors agree that this is the fastest and best treatment for diverticulosis. Fiber—the indigestible parts of plant foods—keeps stools soft so they pass easily

HERBAL POWER

A Tea to Tame Pain

Here is a potent herbal tea for relieving diverticular symptoms, says David Winston, a founding professional member of the American Herbalists Guild and founder and president of Herbalist and Alchemist in Broadway, New Jersey. It contains plants known to help ease inflammation, spasms, and gas.

Mix equal parts of dried yarrow (*Achillea millefolium*), fennel seed (*Foeniculum vulgare*), dried chamomile (*Matricaria recutita*), and ground and dried wild yam root (*Dioscorea villosa*). Place 2 teaspoons of this mixture in 8 ounces of water, stir, then cover, and let it steep for 1 hour. You can drink up to three cups a day, he says. Be sure to strain the tea before drinking.

through the colon. The trouble is that most people get only half as much fiber as they need. To boost your intake, build your meals around beans, vegetables, and whole grains like brown rice, bulgur, and barley. Eat oatmeal or bran cereal for breakfast. Leave the skins on your fruits and vegetables.

One warning: If you have diverticulitis, don't increase your fiber intake until infections are gone since roughage can be an irritant.

Increase your water intake to eight 8-ounce glasses per day. Lack of liquid is a common reason for hard-to-pass stools, says Andrew T. Weil, M.D., clinical professor of internal medicine and director of the integrative medicine program at the University of Arizona College of Medicine in Tucson and author of *Spontaneous Healing*.

Engage in vigorous activity for 30 to 40 minutes, 3 or 4 days a week. Exercise can relieve abdominal congestion, restore normal bowel movements, and promote blood and lymph circulation needed for cleansing and repairing damaged intestinal tissues. It also helps manage stress, which is widely accepted as a foe to digestive balance. "Walking and any of your favorite vigorous activities are helpful. But my favorite exercise for diverticulitis patients is water aerobics in warm water, which supports joints and promotes bowel regularity," says Nancy Russell, M.D., an internist in Kansas City, Missouri, and a member of the American Holistic Medical Association.

Take one or two "probiotic" capsules with meals. A healthy bowel is populated by beneficial bacteria, or probiotics, that complete the digestion of proteins and carbohydrates while also keeping bad bacteria at bay. "When someone contracts diverticulitis, I usually figure that there is some sort of bacterial imbalance," says William D. Nelson, N.D., a naturopathic physician in Colorado Springs, Colorado. He recommends the probiotics L. acidophilus and Bifidobacterium, which are found in the refrigerated section of most health food stores. Look for a supplement that contains 1.5 billion microorganisms per gram and "fructooligosaccharides" (FOS). This is food for the bacteria that helps them get established in your colon. Take one or two capsules with each meal for 6 months, or until your symptoms are resolved.

Relieve digestive inflammation with Roberts Complex. You can purchase this mix of healing plants at health food stores; follow the instructions on the label. "It's a classic remedy among naturopaths," says Dr. Nelson. Look for a brand that contains marsh mallow, slippery elm, goldenseal, echinacea, cabbage powder, and bromelain. Take the formula for 3 months, or until your symptoms are resolved.

Enlist five pancreatic enzymes to aid digestion. Look for a formula at the health food store that contains lipase to digest fat and oils, cellulase to digest fiber, amylase to digest starch and sugar, lactase to digest milk, and protease for protein, advises Dr. Russell. Take it according to the package directions for as long as needed.

Other Approaches

Have 2 teaspoons of aloe vera juice two times a day, straight or in tea or juice. Sold in health food stores, the juice of aloe is well-known for healing irritation of the gastrointestinal tract. It is also helpful as a mild laxative, explains Dr. Russell.

Take two tablets of B-complex 50 twice a day. The B vitamins are powerful nutrients for the colon and might also ease stress, says Dr. Russell. She also recommends, if possible, supplementing with 500 to 2,000 milligrams of vitamin C a day as well as 400 to 600 international units (IU) of vitamin E and 10,000 to 15,000 IU of vitamin A.

Take 40 to 80 milligrams a day of ginkgo (*Ginkgo biloba*) capsules. Be sure to get a variety containing 24 percent ginkgo flavone glycosides. Most people know ginkgo for improving memory and alertness. But since ginkgo helps microcirculation, it may help reestablish the tiny blood vessels in the gastrointestinal tract, explains Dr. Nelson. Take ginkgo all the while you are trying to heal your gastrointestinal tract, typically 6 months.

Stimulate digestion and relieve constipation with bitter herbs. Put 10 to 15 drops of Angostura bitters in a shot glass of your favorite tea or juice and drink it before meals, advises David Winston, a founding professional member of the American Herbalists Guild and founder and president of Herbalist and Alchemist in Broadway, New Jersey. Angostura bitters are made from the herb gentian and can be purchased at grocery and liquor stores. Other beneficial bitters include dandelion, endive, radicchio, and broccoli rabe. You may also like drinking chicory, a healthy coffee substitute.

Relieve tension by giving your breathing attention. Negative emotions result in negative effects on your bowels, says Joel Fuhrman, M.D., director of the Amwell Health Center in Belle Mead, New Jersey, and author of *Fasting and Eating for Health*.

Bringing focus to your breathing is a natural tranquilizer for the nervous system, explains Dr. Weil. Try his simple relaxation technique: Start seated with your back straight. Place the tip of your tongue just behind your upper front teeth, and keep it there for the entire exercise. Making a "whoosh" sound, exhale completely through your mouth. Now inhale quietly through your nose to the count of four. Next, hold your breath for a count of seven. Exhale completely through your mouth, making a "whoosh" sound, to a count of eight. Repeat this cycle three more times for a total of four breaths. Do this at least twice a day, with progressively slower breathing counts.

Consider going on a short, doctor-approved fast to help the digestive system get back on track. When people are hospitalized with diverticulitis, they are put on liquid diets, which are, essentially, fasts. Applied to hundreds of conditions, fasting, when done correctly, enhances the body's ability to heal itself, says Dr. Fuhrman.

Avoiding food gives the colon an opportunity to rest. Fasting also gives beneficial bacteria a chance to repopulate themselves, Dr. Fuhrman explains. Do a home fast only under the supervision of your doctor, he cautions.

Dry Hair

Each strand of hair is wrapped in a protective shield made of transparent overlapping fibers. These fibers seal in moisture, protect the hair shaft from exposure, and give your tresses their healthy, glowing sheen.

If you strip away that moisture with excessive sun exposure, daily shampooing, blow-drying, and hair dyes, the fibrous coat of armor cracks, splits, and peels away, leaving your crowning glory dry and brittle.

The Blended Prescription

Note: To learn about cautions and possible side effects of the remedies in this chapter, see page 253.

Unusually dry, coarse, or brittle hair may be a sign that your thyroid gland isn't producing enough hormone. If you think this could be the cause of your hair problems, see your doctor. But in most cases, it is merely abuse that is causing your hair to frizzle. So get it out of the sun, quit using so many chemicals on it, and try these three steps to help restore the natural moisture, as prescribed by our blended-medicine experts.

For immediate relief, switch to a shampoo and conditioner specially formulated for dry hair. Salon-quality shampoos and conditioners lubricate and help repair the hair shaft, says Michael Traub, N.D., a naturopathic physician in Kailua Kona, Hawaii. Herbal shampoos and conditioners for dry hair are also available at health food stores.

For longer-term relief, take 1 tablespoon daily of one of the following: flaxseed (*Linum usitatissimum*) oil, evening primrose (*Oenothera biennis*) oil, borage (*Borago officinalis*) oil, or omega-3 fish oil. Or take 3,000 to 5,000 milligrams of one of these oils in capsule form each day, says William

D. Nelson, N.D., a naturopathic physician in Colorado Springs, Colorado. These oils, called essential fatty acids, can restore the natural oils in your hair and promote healthier cells and hair follicles. Note that it could take up to 3 months for this to take effect, so be patient.

Provide your hair follicles with good nutritional support. Take the following vitamins and minerals, recommends Chris Meletis, N.D., professor of natural pharmacology and nutrition, dean of clinical education, and chief medical officer at the National College of Naturopathic Medicine in Portland, Oregon.

Vitamin A: 5,000 to 10,000 international units (IU) per day

Vitamin E: 400 to 800 IU per day

Zinc: 30 to 50 milligrams per day

Earache

There are three primary causes for ear pain: pressure inside the ear, infection, or sudden changes in external air pressure that wrench the eardrum out of position.

Often, nasal congestion is behind those first two causes. When you have a cold, the narrow canal leading from your nose to the middle ear—the Eustachian tube—gets dammed up, and the pain comes from internal fluids trying to get past. Or you have mucus or pus gathering behind your eardrum; as pressure builds, the pain starts pounding.

What would cause an earache-inducing change in air pressure? Well, most common are flying (particularly taking off and landing), scuba diving, and riding a high-speed elevator to the 110th floor of the World Trade Center.

The Blended Prescription

Note: To learn about cautions and possible side effects of the remedies in this chapter, see page 253.

See your doctor if you have severe pain, discharge, hearing loss, an earache accompanied by a fever of 102°F or above, or tenderness in the soft areas near your ear, jaw, or upper neck.

For air travelers, see a doctor if during a flight you feel acute pain that doesn't go away immediately afterward, since that could be a sign of a perforated eardrum. For swimmers, see a doctor if you have persistent itching and discomfort from swimmer's ear that doesn't go away when you try the vinegar-and-alcohol solution offered on page 86.

But what if the earache isn't all that bad, and you suspect you can clear it up with home remedies? Here is a six-step prescription from our blended-medicine experts.

Make herbal ear drops. Place three drops of garlic (*Allium sativum*) oil and two drops of mullein (*Verbascum thapsus*) oil directly into the aching ear. Do this three or four times a day until the pain subsides. Garlic and mullein are good bacteria fighters, and garlic also helps boost immunity.

To help fight the germs causing the pain and pressure, supplement with daily doses of immune-stimulating herbs. Take up to 1,200 milligrams of echinacea (*Echinacea purpurea*) in three to six divided doses; 1,800 milligrams of goldenseal (*Hydrastis canadensis*) in three divided doses, but not for more than a week; and up to 5 milligrams of fresh allicin, the active ingredient in garlic (look for a garlic supplement that says "fresh" on the label).

Boost your daily intake of immunity-bolstering vitamins and minerals. Here are the four best to take.

Vitamin C: Up to 4,000 milligrams per day in divided doses

Vitamin A: 50,000 international units (IU) each day for 2 days, followed by 5,000 IU per day for up to 4 weeks

Zinc: Up to 100 milligrams per day

Copper: 4 milligrams per day

Try Chamomilla 30C and Belladonna 6C, two homeopathic remedies. Be sure to follow the directions on the labels.

Treat swimmer's ear with a mixture of vinegar and alcohol. Mix ½ ounce of distilled white vinegar with ½ ounce of rubbing alcohol and put three drops of the mixture in the affected ear three times daily until the pain subsides. The alcohol helps evaporate any remaining water drops, and vinegar kills lingering bacteria.

Apply heat to the ear to promote healing bloodflow. Heat a water bottle, towel, or heating pad wrapped in a towel to a comfortably hot level and apply to your ear for 20 minutes or until the pain goes away, whichever comes first.

Other Approaches

Take all reasonable steps to reduce nasal congestion. By keeping your sinuses clear, you help relieve pressure inside your eardrums and prevent blockages inside the Eustachian tubes. Solutions for unclogging your nose include using a plain saline nasal spray two or three times a day; eating spicy, peppery foods; and, if necessary, using a decongestant according to the package instructions.

Use essential oils to prevent earache. Combine two or three drops of the essential oil of immortelle (*Helichrysum italicum*), also known as everlasting, with two or three drops of the essential oil of lavender (*Lavandula vera*) or with one drop of the essential oil of damask rose (*Rosa damascena*), and add them to an ounce of sweet almond or vegetable oil. Dip two cotton balls in the mixture and gently place one in each ear, says Mark Stengler, N.D., a naturopathic physician in Carlsbad, California, and author of *The Natural Physician*. Then spread some oil on your fingers and massage the ear and the skin around it, he says. These oils help prevent infection.

Note: See your doctor before using an herbal ear preparation if you already have ear pain or if there is a discharge.

Make a drinkable herbal juice with 30 drops of echinacea (*Echinacea purpurea*) tincture and 30 drops of goldenseal (*Hydrastis canadensis*) tincture in juice or water. Echinacea strengthens immunity by stimulating white blood cell production, while goldenseal harbors antibacterial compounds, says Michael Traub, N.D., a naturopathic physician in Kailua Kona, Hawaii.

Eczema

An itchy rash appears out of nowhere. You scratch. It itches. You scratch harder. It keeps itching. The skin turns dry, flaky, scaly, and red or black. Blisters sometimes pop up, and they itch, too.

Eczema, or atopic dermatitis, is an inflammatory skin allergy that can surface on your neck, face, and legs and within the folds of your elbows, knees, and wrists. Food allergies and stress are among the top contributors to the problem. Laundry detergents, harsh soaps, rough and scratchy clothing, dust, pollen, and the dry, cold winter months can also trigger a flare-up.

The Blended Prescription

Note: To learn about cautions and possible side effects of the remedies in this chapter, see page 253.

See your doctor if the eczema is very red, causes severe pain, or drains pus or if you have a fever—all of these are signs of infection. To stop the deep, painful itching, you need to pinpoint what is causing it and incorporate some dietary changes. Here is a seven-step prescription from our blended-medicine experts to get you started.

If the itching is intense, reach for a 1 percent hydrocortisone cream at your local drugstore. Hydrocortisone creams should quickly soothe the itching and reduce inflammation. Apply a thin layer four times a day.

Take two pellets of the homeopathic remedy Sulfur 6C every 15 minutes for four doses, followed by two pellets

---

HERBAL POWER

A Tea for Skin

In a nonaluminum pot, combine 2 tablespoons each of dried licorice (*Glycyrrhiza glabra*), burdock (*Arctium lappa*), and dandelion root (*Taraxacum officinale*). Pour 3 cups of water into the pot. Cover tightly and bring the water to a boil. Let simmer for 15 to 20 minutes. (If the liquid reduces too much, add enough water so that you end up with three cups of tea.) Strain and drink.

These herbs improve liver function to help your body eliminate toxins, says William D. Nelson, N.D., a naturopathic physician in Colorado Springs, Colorado. They also correct hormonal imbalances and contain anti-inflammatory and anti-allergenic properties to prevent eczema and promote healthier skin. To get the most benefit, drink the tea three times a day.

every 4 hours until the itching subsides. Then reduce the dose to two pellets four times a day until the rash heals completely. This remedy is especially good if your skin is dry, rough, red, and itchy. Other possible homeopathic remedies include Petroleum 6C, Rhus tox. 6C, or Graphites 6C, all taken as directed above.

Take the following vitamins, minerals, and supplements for relief from eczema.

Vitamin A: 5,000 to 10,000 international units (IU) per day. Vitamin A promotes healthy skin.

Vitamin C: 1,000 milligrams per day. This vitamin acts as a natural antihistamine to reduce inflammation.

Zinc: 45 to 60 milligrams per day. Zinc has antioxidant properties and is necessary for wound healing and collagen formation, which supports the skin. Take zinc in three divided doses with meals to avoid nausea.

Quercetin: 500 milligrams per day. Quercetin is a bioflavonoid found in fruits and vegetables that is available in supplement form. It is believed to battle allergic reactions and reduce inflammation.

Each day, take 1½ tablespoons of one of the following: flaxseed (*Linum usitatissimum*) oil, evening primrose (*Oenothera biennis*) oil, borage (*Borago officinalis*) oil, or omega-3 fish oil. Or take 3,000 to 5,000 milligrams of one of these oils in capsule form each day, says William D. Nelson, N.D., a naturopathic physician in Colorado Springs, Colorado. These oils, called essential fatty acids, play a significant role in preventing allergies and inflammation, he says. Most people with eczema have low levels.

Pour ⅔ cup of Epsom salts into a tub filled 3 to 5 inches deep with warm water, and soak in it for 20 to 30 minutes. This is a good soother if eczema affects multiple areas of your body. The Epsom salts help detoxify your body, soften your skin, and make it less scaly and less likely to crack or bleed, says Jennifer Brett, N.D., a naturopathic physician in Norwalk and Stratford, Connecticut.

Mix 15 drops of chickweed (*Stellaria media*) tincture in a 2-inch dollop of moisturizing cream. Rub the mixture into the affected area, says Michael Traub, N.D., a naturopathic physician in Kailua Kona, Hawaii. Chickweed soothes itches, he says. For the best results, use the mixture within 3 minutes after you bathe.

Launch an allergy-elimination diet to identify or rule out foods that may be causing the eczema. How? Stop eating dairy products, eggs, peanuts, wheat, and meat for 10 days. Then reintroduce them one at a time every 3 days. That way, you will know which food to blame if you develop a reaction. Most people with eczema are allergic to all or some of these foods.

Eyestrain

Think of your eyes as a set of delicate but powerful muscles that work nonstop 17 to 18 hours a day. Like other parts of your body, your eye muscles are susceptible to stress and overuse. When you focus intently on a book or computer screen, your brain sends constant messages to your optic nerve to stay alert and keep the object in focus. Heeding the call, your eye muscles work valiantly to maintain sharp images. But when they don't get relief, your eyesight can blur from the strain.

The Blended Prescription

Note: To learn about cautions and possible side effects of the remedies in this chapter, see page 253.

SKILLFUL HEALERS

Behavioral Optometry

If you must do a lot of close work, consider going to a behavioral optometrist for a pair of occupational glasses. With these specially fitted glasses, your lenses are matched to the task you perform most often, says Paul Planer, O.D., a behavioral optometrist in Atlanta and past president of the International Academy of Sports Vision in Harrisburg, Pennsylvania.

These lenses may also be tinted. "Typically, a light gray tint works best for computer work because it tends to make the letters on the computer screen come out a bit and offer more contrast," Dr. Planer says. To find a behavioral optometrist, contact the Optometric Extension Program Foundation in Santa Ana, California.

Maybe your eyes just need downtime to help ease the strain. Or they might need a more eye-friendly environment. But when eyestrain sneaks up, there are some easy remedies to bring relief. Here is a six-step prescription from our blended-medicine experts to set your sights on.

Take a break from your close-up work. "It's not natural for our eyes to focus on a two-dimensional plane like a computer screen without straining," says Paul Planer, O.D., a behavioral optometrist in Atlanta and past president of the International Academy of Sports Vision in Harrisburg, Pennsylvania. (A behavioral optometrist approaches and treats the eye as part of the whole body system.) Whether you are gazing at a monitor or the pages of a book, look away every 15 minutes, he recommends. Close your eyes for 10 to 20 seconds while breathing deeply and slowly.

Also, as part of your eye-relief break, stand up and do a

body stretch. With that movement, you relieve your eyes from their focusing work and get more blood and oxygen circulating, says Dr. Planer.

Blink frequently. "Blinking distributes new tears across the corners of your eyes, which keeps them healthy and moist," says Bob Lee, O.D., assistant professor of optometry and coordinator of computer vision services at Southern California College of Optometry in Fullerton. That action maintains optical clarity and reduces eye dryness.

Shield your eyes from glaring light, and change any flickering ones. Reflection from a monitor hastens eyestrain, cautions Dr. Planer. Change the position of the monitor or use lower-intensity room lighting. If fluorescent lights are flickering, change them to head off headaches and eyestrain, he advises.

Apply moist compresses over your closed eyes. Twice a day, close your eyes, tilt back your head, and place a warm washcloth over your eyelids for a few minutes. A cool compress moistened with raspberry-leaf tea (*Rubus idaeus*) also may bring relief. After removing the compress, gently massage your eyelids for 10 to 15 minutes. The warm moisture rejuvenates and relaxes tired eyes and unclogs pores.

Take eyebright. During intense eye use, take this herb (*Euphrasia officinalis*) as a tea two or three times a day.

Take 10,000 international units (IU) of vitamin A each day. Vitamin A has long been associated with eye health, and a deficiency has been shown to increase the likelihood of eye problems.

Other Approaches

Every 15 minutes, focus on various objects at different distances. For computer users, look away from your computer screen and focus on an object that's farther away— a clock on the wall or cars passing outside your window, suggests Dr. Planer. "Also try to vary the distance of your computer screen—move back a few inches if you have a movable keyboard," he says.

Take a 30C dose of the homeopathic remedy Ruta, also called Ruta graveolens, two times a day, when you are feeling symptoms of eyestrain. "Ruta is the number one homeopathic treatment for eyestrain because it relaxes the eye muscles with no side effects," says Mark Stengler, N.D., a naturopathic physician in Carlsbad, California, and author of *The Natural Physician*. Let the pellets dissolve in your mouth, he advises.

Fatigue

Fatigue is perhaps one of the most common ailments, varying from mild and intermittent to chronic and severe. Often, it is the result of subtle chemical imbalances involving hormones and the "messenger" molecules that connect body and mind, says Keith Berndtson, M.D., an integrative medicine specialist at American WholeHealth Centers in Chicago.

When is fatigue healthy? When it is the natural result of a physically and mentally active day. But if poor living habits, improper diet, chronic sleep deprivation, excess stress, depression, or illness is causing you to feel fatigued, then the toll on your health may already be considerable.

The Blended Prescription

Note: To learn about cautions and possible side effects of the remedies in this chapter, see page 253.

Fatigue can be a sign of many illnesses, including anemia or thyroid, adrenal, liver, or kidney problems. You will need to get a doctor's advice if you have been so constantly tired for 2 weeks or more that you can't do your normal activities. But if your fatigue seems to be temporary, here is a five-step prescription from our blended-

---

Alexander Technique

This is a method for improving your posture and correcting some of the ways you might "misuse" your body when you are engaged in daily activities. The technique increases your awareness of what muscles you are overusing and those you are underusing. Both situations can cause muscle fatigue and lead to chronic pain. After mastering this technique, you will have more energy while going about your normal activities, says Laura Smith, a certified teacher of the Alexander Technique in Brooklyn, New York.

An Alexander Technique instructor will work with you in a series of private sessions that usually last 30 to 45 minutes. The teacher evaluates how you stand, sit, walk, and do other ordinary movements. Using a light touch and verbal instruction, he'll help you recognize and change inefficient habits and find new resources of energy. For instance, while you sit and stand, the instructor will place a hand on various muscle groups that are overworking and need release. With the instructor's guidance, you learn to move without taxing your back, neck, and shoulder muscles. For a list of certified instructors in your area, write to the North American Society of Teachers of the Alexander Technique at 3010 Hennepin Avenue South, Suite 10, Minneapolis, MN 55408.

medicine experts to boost energy, concentration, and motivation.

First and foremost, check your diet and sleeping patterns. More than almost anything else, neglecting these two factors can trigger tiredness. So, if you have been skipping meals or consistently eating low-nutrient foods, healthier eating patterns might remedy your fatigue. Likewise, if you have been cutting back on sleep, granting yourself a full 8 hours each night might solve the problem. The test of a good night's sleep? If you can get up without a struggle in the morning, you have found the right sleep pattern.

Every day, take a multivitamin/mineral supplement to make sure that your body has all the ingredients it needs for energy. Here is the proper mix, says Paula G. Maas, D.O., M.D., a homeopathic doctor and chairman of primary care at the Touro University College of Osteopathic Medicine in San Francisco.

Vitamin B_{12}: 250 to 2,000 micrograms. This B vitamin, along with the next two, helps keep your metabolism revved up.

Folic acid: 400 micrograms

Pantothenic acid: 100 to 200 milligrams

Vitamin C: 1,000 to 3,000 milligrams. Vitamin C helps support your adrenal glands.

Chromium: 200 micrograms. This mineral stabilizes blood sugar and boosts metabolism.

Zinc and iron: Make sure that these two are in your supplement. Both are essential fatigue-fighters.

In addition to your multivitamin, supplement your diet with 800 milligrams of magnesium glycinate. Research has shown that people with chronic fatigue have lower levels of magnesium in their blood. Magnesium supplements appear to provide some relief by improving stamina and endurance.

Look for an herbal naturopathic remedy labeled as an adrenal-support combination, such as Adren-Comp Herbal Complex capsules. It likely will contain vitamin B₅, Siberian ginseng (*Eleutherococcus senticosus*), Asian ginseng (*Panax ginseng*), and licorice (*Glycyrrhiza glabra*).

Enroll in a tai chi or yoga class. These disciplines teach tension-releasing, body-invigorating stretches and positions that have thousands of years of therapeutic history.

Other Approaches

Rise at the same time on weekends. Sleeping late on the weekends can make getting up on Monday torture, says Suzan Jaffe, Ph.D., associate adjunct professor of psychiatry and nursing at the University of Miami in Florida. It is okay to deviate a little—by an hour or so. But if you stay on a regular sleep/wake schedule, you will probably feel less tired.

Mist yourself with peppermint water. The smell of peppermint seems to have the ability to motivate us to action, says Brigitte Mars, a professional member of the American Herbalists Guild and a clinical herbalist with UniTea Herbs in Boulder, Colorado. To benefit, add 15 drops of peppermint (*Mentha piperita*) essential oil to an 8-ounce spray bottle of water. Spray your face and the air around you (with your eyes and mouth closed) whenever you start to drag, she suggests.

Rub your feet for a few minutes whenever you feel tired. "Any kind of strong foot massage will help energize someone who is feeling a little tired," says Mary Muryn, a certified reflexology instructor from Westport, Connecticut. Use the thumbs of both hands (or the eraser end of a pencil) to knead the very center of the bottom of your bare foot for a few minutes. You can also firmly roll your

HERBAL POWER

Go with Ginseng

Asian ginseng (*Panax ginseng*) and Siberian ginseng (*Eleutherococcus senticosus*) are reportedly superstar herbs when it comes to boosting energy and improving concentration. Russian cosmonauts and Asian athletes use the ginsengs to better cope with stress. These herbs are reported to improve alertness and immunity, says James A. Duke, Ph.D., a botanical consultant, a former ethnobotanist with the U.S. Department of Agriculture who specializes in medicinal plants, and author of *The Green Pharmacy.*

You can drink ginseng as a tea or take it in capsule form. For tea, put about 1 teaspoon of ginseng in a cup of boiling water. Let it steep for 5 minutes or so. Strain and drink. Stick to one cup a day, Dr. Duke says. If you want to take capsules, follow the specific dosage directions on the product you buy. You may need to take ginseng for a month or more before you see results.

foot back and forth on a specially designed foot roller. If you don't have a foot roller, just use a glass soft-drink bottle, suggests Muryn. If you tip it on its side, you can roll it back and forth with your foot, putting pressure on the sole. If foot massage is a problem, rub the center of your hand with the opposite thumb or a pencil eraser.

Eat barley grass or wheat grass daily. Available in some organic supermarkets, these grasses can be added to salads, says Mars. You can also buy barley grass or wheat grass juice. They are full of fatigue-fighting B vitamins and iron. Add ½ cup to your salad or drink 8 ounces a day to help get rid of fatigue, recommends Mars.

Avoid caffeine and high-sugar junk foods. Caffeine and the sugar in junk foods may give you an initial energy boost, says Dr. Berndtson. But after a few hours, you will crash and feel even more tired than before.

Exercise at least three times a week for 30 minutes or more. Though it sounds contradictory, spending energy is sometimes the best way to get it. If you end up feeling even more tired when you have been lying on the couch, go for more activity, suggests Dr. Berndtson. In as little as a week or two, you will probably begin to have more pep.

Flatulence

When you eat or drink, you often swallow air. As it enters your stomach and weaves its way through the intestines, the gas is too much to absorb. So the overload leaves the rectum in the form of flatulence.

Undigested food in the small intestine can also create flatulence. As food travels into your large intestine, bacteria work hard to break it down. And as the food ferments, it releases hydrogen, carbon dioxide, and, occasionally, methane and sulfur gases (which give flatulence its odor). The foul-smelling odor that floats out of the rectum is the by-product of overindustrious bacteria going about their good work.

The Blended Prescription

Note: To learn about cautions and possible side effects of the remedies in this chapter, see page 253.

Most people pass gas about 14 times a day, so there is nothing abnormal about the process. But not all flatulence problems are alike. If you have sharp pain or tenderness in your abdomen, see a doctor.

Here are prescriptions for dealing with short- and long-term gas problems, as prescribed by our blended-medicine experts. For acute or severe gas pains, try the following strategies.

Do some abdominal crunches to help move the gas through your system. To do the crunches, lie on your back with your fingertips cupped behind your ears, your knees bent at a 45-degree angle, and your feet together, flat on the floor, about 6 inches from your buttocks. Use your abdominal muscles to lift your upper torso a few inches, and then slowly lower yourself to the floor. Repeat. Try doing three sets of 10, resting for 15 to 30 seconds between sets.

Rock in a rocking chair or jump on a mini-trampoline. These actions get the gas moving faster through your colon.

Drink an herbal tea to help relieve gas pain. Try chamomile (*Matricaria recutita*), ginger (*Zingiber officinale*), peppermint (*Mentha piperita*), or lemon balm (*Melissa officinalis*).

Have a dose of the homeopathic remedies Lycopodium 6C, Chamomilla 6C, or Nux vomica 6C. Take two pellets every 15 minutes for 1 hour, then two pellets every hour for four doses on the first day. After that, take two pellets four times a day until your symptoms resolve. If your symptoms are severe or persist for many days, see your doctor.

Use over-the-counter remedies, such as Infants' Mylicon Drops (adult dosages are given on the label) or Gas-X. Follow the directions on the package.

When gas is recurrent or persistent, you may need to change your eating habits. Here is a prescription that will help give you long-term relief.

Eat slowly to avoid swallowing too much air with your food.

HERBAL POWER

Fennel for Flatulence

The herb fennel (*Foeniculum vulgare*) contains carminatives, an ingredient proven to expel gas from the intestinal tract, says Andrew T. Weil, M.D., clinical professor of internal medicine and director of the integrative medicine program at the University of Arizona College of Medicine in Tucson and author of *Spontaneous Healing*. He recommends that you chew ½ teaspoon of fennel seeds after meals or whenever you feel bloated from gas. Or drink a cup of fennel-flavored tea after meals.

Test for food sensitivity with an elimination diet. For 3 weeks, give up all dairy, egg, corn, wheat, and citrus foods. If you notice an improvement, add back one food group every 3 to 4 days to see which food brings on symptoms.

For 1 month, try taking regular doses of the digestive enzymes that are available at health food stores. Follow the instructions on the package.

Have 1 tablespoon of acidophilus powder in water each morning. This supplement will help restore normal, "good" bacteria to the digestive tract.

Before you eat gas-producing foods like beans or cabbage, take the over-the-counter enzyme product Beano. Follow the label directions.

Other Approaches

Every 4 hours, take two capsules of activated charcoal. Charcoal helps absorb intestinal gas, says Judyth

Reichenberg-Ullman, N.D., a naturopathic doctor and co-director of the Northwest Center for Homeopathic Medicine in Edmonds, Washington. It is available without prescription in most drugstores.

Begin each morning with a 5-minute gas-releasing stomach massage. Before you rise from bed, lie flat on your back and put your right palm on the lower right side of your belly, just above your pelvic bone, suggests Laura Norman, a licensed massage therapist, a leading reflexology authority in New York City, and author of *Feet First: A Guide to Foot Reflexology*. Knead that spot with your fingertips, pressing firmly. Then slowly move clockwise, stopping at the five, eight, and one o'clock spots on your abdomen area to knead in circular motions with your fingers. "This massage helps to get things moving along inside your digestive tract," says Norman.

Flu

Each year, the flu virus goes on the prowl, and every few years, this predatory virus has a new form. Unless you have been inoculated, your body is a relatively easy target for infection.

Once these viruses latch on to the mucous membranes in your nose or mouth, a fierce battle ensues. Attempting to rid itself of the virus, your body heats up like a furnace, becomes inflamed in certain places, and produces mucus. Actually, it is by these healthy responses that miserable symptoms appear. Headache, fatigue, muscle aches, chills, sore throat, and congestion all reflect that the body is trying to kill the virus.

The Blended Prescription

Note: To learn about cautions and possible side effects of the remedies in this chapter, see page 253.

The best defense is a great offense: Get a flu shot each year. For healthy young adults, it is 70 to 90 percent effective against the most common strains of the disease, which change each year. Even when it doesn't provide full protection, your symptoms are likely to be less severe if you've had the vaccine. The best time to get your annual shot is October or early November.

If the flu does hit, symptoms should dissipate within 7 days. If you are getting weaker, sustaining a temperature above 101°F, or coughing from deep in your chest, see a doctor. Pneumonia could be developing.

Here is a seven-step prescription to end a bout with a flu as fast as possible, as prescribed by our experts in blended medicine.

Take up to 1,000 milligrams of acetaminophen every 4 hours. This will reduce aches and bring down any fever.

Drink, sip, and guzzle fluids—water, juice, soup, tea, and broth—as often as possible, all day long. These help keep virus-fighting mucus thin and flowing. While you have the flu, you should get 10 eight-ounce glasses of fluids a day (and don't count soda or coffee).

Among your fluid intake should be several cups a day of herbal tea. Elder flower (*Sambucus canadensis*) and licorice (*Glycyrrhiza*, various species), for example, are great for their capacity to stimulate your immune system. In addition, warm liquids are soothing for the body, prevent viruses from reproducing, and even have a mild decongestant effect. Two teaspoons of these dry herbs, steeped for 10 minutes, will bring out all their medicinal qualities. Strain before drinking.

HERBAL POWER

Soothe with Ginger

Sip a cup of hot ginger tea to boost your immune system's fighting power. Ginger (*Zingiber officinale*) is full of antiviral compounds to help fight infection, reduce pain and fever, and suppress coughing. "Ginger heats up the body, making it very difficult for viruses to survive," says Ellen Evert Hopman, a master herbalist in Amherst, Massachusetts; a professional member of the American Herbalists Guild; and author of *Tree Medicine, Tree Magic*. What's more, it is a natural expectorant and a mild sedative that will help you rest.

Chop a 1-inch piece of fresh ginger into slivers. Place them in a nonaluminum pot and add 2 cups of water. Cover tightly, simmer for 20 minutes, then strain into a cup. Squeeze in the juice of half a lemon. Add honey to taste.

Drink no more than two cups a day, says Hopman. "Too much can irritate the lungs and actually produce mucus."

Use three vitamins to give your immune system a jump start.

Beta-carotene: 25,000 international units (IU) four times a day for 5 days. This will enhance your immune response, as numerous studies have shown.

Vitamin C: 2,000 milligrams three times a day. This vitamin is a natural antihistamine and helps fight viruses.

Vitamin E: 400 IU twice a day. This vitamin helps fight free radicals, which are produced when your immune system is under attack.

Every 2 to 3 hours, suck on a 15-milligram zinc glu-conate lozenge (like Cold-Eeze). Studies show that zinc can help cut the length of a cold or flu by more than half. Lozenges particularly help battle coughing and congestion.

Take supplements of an immune-bolstering herb. Try goldenseal (*Hydrastis canadensis*), echinacea (*Echinacea*, various species), or astragalus (*Astragalus*, various species). Take 200 milligrams of any one of these four times a day, for up to 7 days.

Finally, take the homeopathic flu product Oscillococcinum, following the instructions on the package. This remedy is available in some drugstores and health food stores.

Other Approaches

Make an aromatic "flu rub." At the first sign of flu symptoms, try this soothing mixture recommended by Susanne Wissell, a licensed massage therapist and principal of the Center for Holistic Botanical Studies in Westford, Massachusetts. Pour 1 ounce of vegetable or almond oil into a small container. Add 11 drops each of eucalyptus (*Eucalyptus radiata*) and ravensara (*Ravensara aromatica*) essential oils, along with 2 drops of cinnamon leaf (*Cinnamomum zeylanicum*) essential oil. Mix well, using a dropper to stir. Then put some drops on your hands and rub the mixture onto your throat and upper chest area. Repeat this treatment throughout the day, suggests Wissell.

You can also apply this blend all over your body at nighttime. "Put on an old pair of pajamas that you don't mind getting some oil on, and get into bed. By the next morning, you should feel fine," says Wissell. Eucalyptus is

SKILLFUL HEALERS

Naturopathy

See a naturopath if you want to consider an intravenous shot of immune-bolstering vitamins and minerals. Called a Meyers cocktail, this nutrient-dense mix contains 500 milligrams of vitamin C, 250 to 500 milligrams of magnesium, 250 to 500 milligrams of calcium, and 50 to 100 milligrams of B-complex vitamins, says Keith Berndtson, M.D., an integrative medicine specialist at American WholeHealth Centers in Chicago.

"Because the vitamins and minerals go straight into your bloodstream, they get pushed right into the cells much more efficiently than if you were to load up on these nutrients orally," says Dr. Berndtson. The immune system boost can last for several hours and even days.

a natural antiseptic, antibacterial, and antiviral oil; ravensara has abundant antiviral compounds; and cinnamon leaf harbors anti-infection and antiviral properties, she says.

Note: Don't use cinnamon bark oil as a substitute for the cinnamon leaf oil.

Eat leafy dark greens and deep orange vegetables. These bolster the immune system so that you can fight off infection, says Maureen Williams, N.D., a naturopathic physician at the New England Center for Integrative Health in Hanover, New Hampshire. Shiitake mushrooms, beets, garlic, and onions are also immunity boosters, she says. "Also try miso soup, found in most health food stores. Miso replaces electrolytes lost through sweating and diarrhea."

Avoid high-carbohydrate foods. Sugar and high-carbohydrate foods such as breads and pasta made with refined white flour, white rice, pretzels, and rice cakes weaken the immune system, says Dr. Williams. Sugar-laden fruit juices are just as guilty.

Skip caffeine and alcohol. When you have the flu, caffeine and alcohol "are rocket fuel for bacteria growth," says Keith Berndtson, M.D., an integrative medicine specialist at American WholeHealth Centers in Chicago. "They create sugar swings in the bloodstream that throw off your immune system response to infections."

Ask your doctor about amantadine or rimantadine. The antiviral prescription drugs amantadine (Amantadine HCl) and rimantadine (Flumadine) can shorten the duration of influenza type A infection. They have also proved 70 to 90 percent effective when used as a type A preventive. Most important, they can also prevent you from developing serious complications such as pneumonia, Reye's syndrome, and convulsions. So be sure to ask your doctor about these antivirals if you are age 65 or older or if you have heart, lung, or kidney disease, diabetes, or another high-risk condition.

Food Poisoning

Food—particularly meat, poultry, and seafood—makes a fine home for bacteria or viruses when it's left in the open air or on microbe-laden surfaces. When you eat tainted food or drink, these powerful organisms seek hideaways in the linings of your stomach and intestines, where they can grow. Once alerted, your immune system responds to engulf the invaders. As this struggle ensues, you experience nausea, abdominal cramps, headache, and possibly vomiting and diarrhea. The symptoms subside once your body overpowers the intruders and breaks down the tainted food.

The Blended Prescription

Note: To learn about cautions and possible side effects of the remedies in this chapter, see page 253.

See a doctor if your symptoms do not improve after a day or two, if you have diarrhea accompanied by vomiting or fever, or if you have blurry vision or impaired hearing. But to cope with everyday food poisoning, rest, stay near a bathroom, and use this five-step prescription from our blended-medicine experts.

Go easy on your eating. Limit your food intake during the bout to clear liquids like ginger ale, apple juice, and broth and gelatin products like Jell-O. The rule is, if you can see through it, you can consume it.

For nausea and diarrhea, take an over-the-counter stomach soother (such as Pepto-Bismol). Follow the instructions on the package. The remedy soothes the inflamed intestinal lining and blocks the toxin's effect.

Help yourself to herbal teas as long as they don't upset your stomach. These include ginger (*Zingiber officinale*), cinnamon (*Cinnamomum zeylanicum*), and chamomile (*Matricaria recutita*).

Take two 100-milligram ginger (*Zingiber officinale*) capsules every 2 to 3 hours. This root herb has a sterling reputation for fighting nausea and soothing the stomach as well as boosting the immune system's ability to fight infection.

Have a homeopathic remedy. Take Arsenicum album 6C for nausea with diarrhea, Ipecacuanha 6C for sudden nausea and vomiting, or Nux vomica 6C for nausea and diarrhea caused by overindulgence in alcohol or food. Take two pellets every 15 minutes for four doses, then two pellets every hour for four doses the first day. After that, take two pellets four times a day until your symptoms are gone.

Foot Pain

The causes of foot pain come in three main varieties: blisters, corns, and bunions. Blisters usually are caused by the intense friction that your foot endures from a new pair of shoes. As the top layer of skin is tugged by unfamiliar footwear, it separates from the closely packed cells on the second layer, and fluid fills the ensuing gap.

Corns have a similar cause: These little balls of dead skin build up over an area that is repeatedly abused, often by shoes that are too tight. They frequently form on the outside of the little toe or the tops of toes, with a nucleus that roots into the skin, pressing on nerve endings.

Finally, a bunion is a little knob that juts out from the base of the big toe. If you wear narrow shoes or if your feet have an atypical structure, the large joint of the big toe is pushed outward every time you take a step. The result is a painful, red, swollen protrusion.

The Blended Prescription

Note: To learn about cautions and possible side effects of the remedies in this chapter, see page 253.

If painful feet prevent you from going about your normal business, see your doctor. You may need to have specially designed orthotics or minor surgery. To take care of minor foot pain on your own, the first step is finding comfortable shoes that fit properly and look good enough to wear every day. That solved, the next step is to take care of the blisters, corns, or bunions that are taking all the bounce from your stride. Here are six steps to consider, as provided by our experts in blended medicine.

Protect areas that shoes rub. If you suspect that a pair of shoes will create a blister by the end of the day, protect the spot with paper tape or first-aid tape that breathes, says Dale Anderson, M.D., clinical assistant professor at the University of Minnesota Medical School in Minneapolis and author of *Muscle Pain Relief in 90 Seconds: The Fold and Hold Method*. Use a few drops of benzoin (*Lindera benzoin*) tincture to help make the tape stick better and toughen the skin, he adds. If you don't have tape, rub petroleum jelly on the spot that is likely to blister to reduce friction.

Wrap corns in moleskin. To protect corns from enduring more friction, protect them with moleskin, advises Steven Subotnick, D.P.M., N.D., Ph.D., clinical professor of biomechanics and surgery at the California College of Podiatric Medicine in Hayward, a specialist in sports medicine, and author of *Sports and Exercise Injuries*. Available in drugstores, moleskin has an adhesive back that sticks to your skin. Take the moleskin off before you go to bed, and put on a fresh piece every morning.

Cover bunions with doughnut pads. A doughnut pad (sometimes labeled a bunion cushion) has a hole cut in the middle to prevent putting pressure on the swollen area. They are available in most drugstores. Some pads have adhesive on the back, while others may need to be adhered with first-aid tape. Position the opening of the pad over the part of your bunion that sticks out the most, says Dr. Subotnick.

At the end of the day, gently massage your feet, then soak them for 15 minutes in Epsom salts. A mixture of magnesium and sulfur, Epsom salts need to be dissolved in warm water. Follow the package directions. An alternative soak is to put a few drops of the essential oils of juniper berry (*Juniperus*, various species) and lavender (*Lavandula officinalis*) in cool water. Continue with massages and soaks as often as necessary to soothe sore feet, says Dr. Subotnick.

Treat blisters, corns, and bunions with nonprescription calendula (*Calendula officinalis*) ointment, a natural antiseptic and anti-inflammatory. Spread the ointment directly on the injured area, even on an open blister, as often as you like, says Stephen Messer, N.D., a naturopathic physician in Eugene, Oregon, and dean of the summer school of the National Center for Homeopathy in Alexandria, Virginia.

Try homeopathic solutions for your feet. You can take these preparations as needed until symptoms resolve themselves. They are all safe to take long-term. You should see results within a couple of weeks.

- For corns, take Ranunculus 6C, two pellets three times a day.
- For calluses, take Lycopodium 6C, two pellets three times a day.
- For a burning feeling, take Sulfur 6C, Graphites 6C, or Apis mellifica 6C, two pellets three times a day.

Other Approaches

Put cotton between your toes to protect the corns that form there. Corns that form between the toes are generally caused by wearing high-heeled shoes, says Dr. Subotnick. A podiatrist may have to trim the corns, but in the meantime, you can buffer them from friction with the cotton balls.

Relax a bunion's tender spot. Put the tip of your middle finger on the underside of the ball of the big toe that has the bunion. Then place the thumb of that hand on the top of the big toe, and gently push and turn the big toe down and under the foot and toward the little toe. "This position will make the bunion look worse but feel better," says Dr. Anderson. Hold that position for at least 90 seconds, then slowly release the toe, repeating several times to help relieve the pain.

Gingivitis

Gingivitis is Latin for "inflamed gums" and is the long-term outcome of food particles lingering in the crevices between the gums and teeth. Left alone, the food helps create invisible slime on teeth called plaque. When calcified plaque builds up around the bases of your teeth, this local irritant inflames gum tissue. While you won't notice gingivitis at its earliest stages, the action of bacteria-fighting white blood cells and plaque may cause your gums to turn red and sore and even to bleed.

The Blended Prescription

Note: To learn about cautions and possible side effects of the remedies in this chapter, see page 253.

You will need the help of a dentist or hygienist to remove plaque that sets up camp around your gum lines. But once your teeth have been professionally cleaned, use this six-step prescription from our blended-medicine experts for returning inflamed gums to health.

Take a high-potency multiple vitamin every day. Getting the vitamins you need improves your health and has a positive effect on your teeth and gums.

Supplement with 1,000 milligrams of vitamin C three times a day until your gums heal. Vitamin C promotes healing of bleeding, unhealthy gums.

Every day, open a vitamin C capsule (any strength) and sprinkle the contents on a soft toothbrush. Brush your gum line with this powder, then rinse.

Make use of a Water Pik or similar cleaning device every day. Clearing out food particles and bacteria helps keep gums healthy.

Floss at least once a day. This simple practice prevents plaque from building up on gums and teeth.

Rinse after every brushing (until your gums get better) with an aloe vera mouthwash that contains no alcohol. Aloe soothes and heals painful gums. You can find aloe vera mouthwashes in health food stores.

Other Approaches

Brush properly to control plaque. Flossing and brushing are the two best ways to reduce the surface film of plaque on your teeth, according to the American Dental Association. Use a soft-bristled brush twice a day, and floss at least daily to clean between your teeth. And don't forget the inside surfaces of your teeth—that is where plaque deposits tend to build up.

Take garlic supplements to help healing and prevent infection. Garlic has a natural antibiotic action, explains Stephen R. Goldberg, D.D.S., a dentist in New York City. Considered the poor man's antibiotic, garlic has often been used to treat infection in Third World countries.

HERBAL POWER

Ease Bleeding with Calendula

Calendula, a type of marigold plant, has properties that heal the mucous membranes. It can also help stop bleeding gums in the case of gingivitis, says Stephen R. Goldberg, D.D.S., a dentist in New York City. He recommends using a nonalcoholic calendula (*Calendula officinalis*) extract. Mix 10 drops of extract in 10 drops of water and use as a mouth rinse twice daily after brushing.

"You could add raw garlic to your meals, but you would have to eat a huge amount to get the same effect," he says. Instead, just take some garlic supplements every day, following the directions on the label.

Try an over-the-counter herbal product to prevent plaque. The herb bloodroot (*Sanguinaria canadensis*) seems to have the amazing ability to prevent bacteria in the mouth from creating plaque, says James A. Duke, Ph.D., a botanical consultant, a former ethnobotanist with the U.S. Department of Agriculture who specializes in medicinal plants, and author of *The Green Pharmacy*. Fortunately, you don't have to forage in the wild for this one. Sanguinarine, the active compound in bloodroot, is an ingredient in an over-the-counter mouthwash called Viadent.

Gout

A big toe. The middle of the night. Those are gout's favorite place and time to strike. Gout, a type of arthritis, occurs when urate crystals concentrate in joints and tendons. Where do these crystals come from? When your body metabolizes a protein called purine, one of the by-products is uric acid. When your kidneys fail to excrete enough uric acid or your body just produces too much of it, it collects and solidifies into urate crystals in the space between the bones and tendons in a joint.

If you have ever had an attack of gout, you know that the symptoms are inflammation, pressure, and some serious pain. In more advanced stages, little urate deposits called tophi can form hard little balls in the hands, feet, or earlobes. Over time, the tophi can cause joint stiffness and deformity. Similar deposits that form in the kidneys can become kidney stones. In severe cases, the excess uric acid can cause your kidneys to deteriorate.

The Blended Prescription

Note: To learn about cautions and possible side effects of the remedies in this chapter, see page 253.

If you play your cards right, you need never have another attack of gout. But if you are in the grips of a current attack, step one is making the pain go away. You should see your doctor if you have severe pain in a joint that persists for more than a few days, especially if you have chills, fever, or red streaks on the skin. Otherwise, here is a six-step prescription for dealing with gout, as recommended by our blended-medicine experts.

Immediately take ibuprofen, following the bottle's directions. This will help reduce the inflammation around affected joints that causes the pain, says Jeffrey R. Lisse, M.D., professor of medicine and director of the division of rheumatology at the University of Texas Medical Branch at Galveston. If the recommended dosage doesn't dent the pain, see your doctor for a stronger painkiller. Do not take aspirin or acetaminophen, because they can make gout worse.

HERBAL POWER

Let Devil's Claw Banish the Evil Pain

Devil's claw (*Harpagophytum procumbens*) works to lower uric acid levels. It also has anti-inflammatory properties, says John Collins, N.D., a naturopathic physician and a teacher of homeopathy at the National College of Naturopathic Medicine in Portland, Oregon. These effects provide a powerful one-two punch against gout. Taking it in tincture form (20 to 30 drops, two or three times a day) can help relieve pain and improve mobility in the joint. Devil's claw is available in health food stores.

To help relieve pain, place an ice compress wrapped in a towel or cloth on the affected area for 20 minutes at a time. You can repeat this process hourly until the pain goes away.

During a gout attack, get plenty of rest and keep the affected joint elevated. Blood and uric acid don't build up and further aggravate the joint in distress when it is elevated, says John Collins, N.D., a naturopathic physician and a teacher of homeopathy at the National College of Naturopathic Medicine in Portland, Oregon.

Try to drink eight 8-ounce glasses of fluids a day. Liquids help dilute uric acid and flush it from your system, says Letitia Watrous, N.D., a naturopathic physician and hydrotherapy specialist at Windrose Naturopathic Clinic in Spokane, Washington. Your best bet is water. Also, watch out for soda and fruit juices that are sweetened with regular sugar or fructose. They can increase uric acid production.

Take 375 milligrams of bromelain at a potency of 2,400 mcu (a standard unit of measurement for enzymes) every 2 to 4 hours between meals. This enzyme, which is derived from pineapples and is available in supplement form, works as an anti-inflammatory to ease the pain of gout, notes Dr. Collins. Take it during an attack and for the 7 to 14 days following. Bromelain starts to

SKILLFUL HEALERS

Hydrotherapy

The ancient practice of hydrotherapy uses water to relieve ailments ranging from headaches to sprained ankles. To treat gout, a hydrotherapist alternates putting terry cloth towels soaked in hot or cold water on the chest and back. The extreme temperature changes increase blood flow through the body, says Letitia Watrous, N.D., a naturopathic physician and hydrotherapy specialist at Windrose Naturopathic Clinic in Spokane, Washington. The blood picks up uric acid and carries it to the kidneys, which dispose of it. The body absorbs about ¼ to ½ cup of water during the treatment, she says. That also helps flush you out because, hydrotherapists think, the water goes right through the pores and tissues, picking up acid and sending it to the kidneys for removal.

"For a patient who has gout in a big toe, we might put painless electrical stimulation through that foot while we are doing the hydrotherapy treatment," says Dr. Watrous. The stimulation greatly increases blood flow through the foot. Most gout patients need only three to five 1-hour therapy sessions, she says. "If they watch their diets, they may not need any kind of medication to be finished with gout for good."

work after a few days, so don't be discouraged if you don't get relief right away. Once it does kick in, brome-lain works better than any other over-the-counter anti-inflammatory, he says. It is available in health food stores.

Drink cherry juice several times every day. It may sound odd, and there is no scientific evidence to back it up, but many people find that drinking cherry juice or eating cherries relieves their gout symptoms, Dr. Collins says. It doesn't matter if the cherries are sweet or sour or if the juice is fresh or canned. It is important, however, to drink only unsweetened juice. Some people have even reported that taking 1 tablespoon of cherry concentrate a day does the trick. You can find this concentrate at health food stores. Likewise, some doctors recommend eating blue-berries for gout relief.

Other Approaches

Eliminate high-purine foods from your diet. "Many people can totally control their gout by eating the right diet," says Dr. Watrous. Eliminate foods that are high in purines so your body doesn't have the raw materials to make urate crystals. Some high-purine foods are organ meats (such as liver and kidney), meats, yeast (brewer's and baking), shellfish, herring, sardines, mackerel, and an-chovies. In addition, reduce the amount of foods you eat that have moderate levels of purines, she says. These in-clude spinach, asparagus, other fish, poultry (especially turkey), and mushrooms.

Avoid alcohol. Alcohol is a double whammy that can often be an outbreak trigger. First, it increases uric acid production by speeding up the breakdown of purines. Second, it slows uric acid excretion. So if you cut down on your alcohol consumption or, better yet, stop drinking alcohol altogether, you might get fantastic relief from gout, says Dr. Watrous.

Eat more whole grains and vegetables. Focusing your diet on whole grains and vegetables and cutting back on simple sugars and saturated fats will also help keep gout at bay, says Dr. Watrous. Simple sugars such as refined sugar, honey, corn syrup, maple syrup, molasses, and fructose increase uric acid production, while saturated fats work to decrease uric acid excretion.

Take 10 to 30 drops of cat's claw (*Uncaria*, various species) tincture three to four times a day. Cat's claw is an herb that can help relieve painful, gouty joints by removing uric acid from the body. It is also an anti-inflammatory, says Dr. Collins. You can buy it in health food stores. Take it for as long as an attack lasts.

Drink 4 to 6 ounces of raw potato juice every hour during an attack. Raw potato juice seems to work as an anti-inflammatory to relieve the pain of gout attacks, says Dr. Collins. You will probably have to make it yourself by putting scrubbed raw potatoes in a juicer. Or you can visit a juice bar; raw potato juice probably isn't a top seller, but the server may make it for you.

Hangover

Alcohol dehydrates you, which makes your cells shrink, then expand, causing a headache and dry mouth. Also, many alcoholic drinks have ingredients, like methanol and acetaldehyde, that cause sick stomachs and headaches in some people. And because alcohol is an anesthetic and a depressant, you may do too much of everything when you are under the influence, and your body pays the price the next day. All these factors contribute to the most notorious of drinkers' woes: hangover.

The Blended Prescription

Note: To learn about cautions and possible side effects of the remedies in this chapter, see page 253.

Hangover is easy to prevent, but by the time you start to dread it, prevention is usually too late. To minimize its effects, take these six actions, as prescribed by our blended-medicine experts.

If you are preparing for bed and still feel the effects of the alcohol you consumed that evening, drink water. The more, the better. Try for at least 12 ounces. The water will help minimize the dehydrating effect of the alcohol.

Before sleep, take 2,000 milligrams of vitamin C and two tablets of B-complex 50. These vitamins may counteract some of the effects of alcohol.

If you have a morning hangover, take two pellets of the homeopathic remedy Nux vomica 6C every 15 minutes until you have had eight doses. Then take two pellets every hour until the hangover ends.

Drink plenty of fresh juices. Best of all is 8 ounces of carrot juice mixed with 2 ounces of beet juice. Drink every 2 hours until your symptoms disappear. The juices rehydrate your body and flush your system of toxins.

Drink herbal tea made from chamomile (*Matricaria recutita*) and white willow (*Salix*, various species). The white willow contains natural salicylates, the active ingredient in aspirin, and the chamomile settles your stomach. Put 1 teaspoon of each herb in a cup, add boiling water, steep for 10 minutes, then strain. Add honey to taste. Drink one cupful three or four times a day as needed.

For headache or pain, take your choice of aceta-minophen, aspirin, or ibuprofen. All may be effective, but aspirin and ibuprofen are harsher on the stomach.

Hay Fever

Histamine, a chemical made by your body's immune system, is normally on your side. It lowers blood pressure, stimulates gastric juices, and helps your circulatory system adapt to cold and heat. But when people with hay fever come into contact with the substances to which they are sensitive, histamines can get overzealous. Since the immune system perceives pollen and other harmless natural material as a threat, it produces a chain reaction of defense mechanisms. The end result is excess histamine, which ultimately causes the all-too-familiar sneezing, runny nose, scratchy throat, congestion, and itchy, watery eyes.

The Blended Prescription

Note: To learn about cautions and possible side effects of the remedies in this chapter, see page 253.

For quick relief, put those renegade histamines in check—then eliminate inflammation, dry up nasal secretions, and clear up watery eyes while encouraging your body to heal itself. Here's a seven-step combination that can make that happen, as prescribed by our blended-medicine experts.

For a hay fever–fighting supplement combination, take 1,000 milligrams of vitamin C and 300 to 500 milligrams of quercetin or mixed bioflavonoids three times a day, along with a once-daily dose of 10,000 international units

HELPFUL HEALERS

Chiropractic

If you visit a chiropractor for neck pain, headaches, or back problems, chances are you may never need to blow your nose in hay fever season.

"We don't know what the underlying mechanism is. But very often, patients come in for one thing and end up having their hay fever problems resolved," says Irwin Heller, D.C., a chiropractic physician at American WholeHealth Centers in Chicago. "By manipulating and adjusting spinal joints to relieve various aches and pains, I've seen nasal congestion as well as other allergy symptoms clear up."

This phenomenon, Dr. Heller says, can be attributed to stimulating the immune system and restoring energy flow through spinal joint manipulation. "We also think that because joint adjustments put you in a totally relaxed state, your body is better able to resist allergens in the air," he says.

(IU) of vitamin A. Vitamin C turbocharges your immune system and reduces histamine release; bioflavonoids are substances in plants available as nutritional supplements that are believed to help fight allergic reactions; vitamin A plays an important role in the health of mucous membranes.

Take two capsules, equivalent to 600 milligrams, of the herb stinging nettle (*Urtica dioica*) three times a day. Studies suggest that stinging nettle provides significant relief from hay fever.

Sip one cup of elder flower (*Sambucus canadensis*) tea three times a day. Elder flower is traditionally used for inflammation of the nasal membrane and contains allergy-wrestling flavonoids. Look for elder flower tea bags at the health food store.

Take two pellets of homeopathic Allium cepa 6C or Euphrasia 6C every 15 minutes for four doses; then two pellets every hour for four doses on your first day. After that, take two pellets four times a day as needed. Allium cepa is made from the plants in the onion family and can relieve classic hay fever symptoms, such as runny nose, cough, and headaches. Euphrasia is the better choice if your eyes are giving you the most trouble.

Pick up some euphorbium homeopathic nasal spray and follow the instructions on the package.

If natural remedies aren't readily available or aren't providing fast relief, turn to the drugstore for an over-the-counter antihistamine (like Benadryl). But be prepared for side effects that include drowsiness, nervousness, gastrointestinal disturbances, insomnia, nausea, and drying of the nose, mouth, and throat.

If even stronger action is needed, you may want to try an over-the-counter anti-allergenic nasal spray such as Nasalcrom. Use as directed on the package. You may also want to seek your doctor's advice about using a prescription steroid nasal spray such as fluticasone (Flonase).

Other Approaches

Add a few drops of eucalyptus (*Eucalyptus globulus*) essential oil to a pan of boiling water, take the pan off the stove, and inhale the steam. This will help open up clogged nasal and bronchial passages. Be careful not to burn yourself by leaning too close to the steam.

Add 2 teaspoons of flaxseed (*Linum usitatissimum*) oil to your diet. Available at health food stores, flaxseed oil is the number one source of essential fatty acids, a vital di-

SKILLFUL HEALERS

Chinese Medicine

Chinese herbs can put an end to seasonal hay fever and perennial allergy symptoms while treating the root of the problem, says Kirk Moulton, a traditional Chinese medicine physician and a certified acupuncturist at American WholeHealth Centers in Chicago.

The tricky part is choosing and finding the right Chinese herb for you and your specific set of symptoms. Since the same Chinese herb can fall under various monikers at health food stores or Asian markets, you need to consult a Chinese medicine practitioner who can tell you exactly what herb you need, how much to take, and for how long.

Depending on your hay fever type and whether it is seasonal or perennial, your doctor may prescribe *Cang Er Zi San* for sneezing and an itchy, runny nose or *Ma Huang Tang* for a stuffy, runny nose, slight headache, and sneezing. *Gan Mao Dan*, a common cold pill, is the Chinese herb that addresses all the classic hay fever symptoms, including an itchy, scratchy throat.

etary supplement that can stave off up to 60 debilitating conditions, including allergies, says David Edelberg, M.D., assistant professor of medicine at Rush Medical College in Chicago and chairman and founder of the American WholeHealth Centers in Chicago, Boston, Denver, and Bethesda, Maryland.

Flaxseed oil helps prevent inflammation of the eyes and nose and other hay fever symptoms. It contains alpha-linolenic acid (an omega-3 fatty acid) and linoleic acid (an omega-6 fatty acid) in huge amounts. If 2 teaspoons of flaxseed oil doesn't sound appetizing, you can take a 1,000-milligram dose in capsule form per day instead.

Pay a visit to an acupuncturist to relieve hay fever symptoms. Acupuncture is one of the best natural medicine therapies for relieving allergies and other upper respiratory illnesses, says Kirk Moulton, a traditional Chinese medicine physician and a certified acupuncturist at American WholeHealth Centers in Chicago. During your visit, expect the doctor to insert needles in strategic points along both sides of your nose to dry up nasal passages and relieve sinus pressure. He may also insert needles in between your eyebrows and in your upper back to strengthen your lungs, says Moulton.

Mix three or four drops each of Roman chamomile (*Chamaemelum nobile*) and lavender (*Lavandula angustifolia*) essential oils with 1 ounce of vegetable oil. Massage your chest and back with this mixture, says Haley Zee, an aromatherapist and president of Haley Zee Associates, an aromatherapy consulting firm and product manufacturer in Leucadia, California. Roman chamomile has strong anti-inflammatory properties to help reduce swelling of nasal and sinus passages. Lavender can also reduce swelling and help dry up nasal secretions.

Take a bath in eucalyptus and other aromatic oils. To tackle the sneezing, runny nose, and itchy, watery eyes, you can use three to five drops of any of the following essential oils: eucalyptus (*Eucalyptus globulus*), lavender (*Lavandula angustifolia*), Roman chamomile (*Chamaemelum nobile*), or rose (*Rosa damascena*).

If you have sensitive skin, first add the drops to ½ cup of grapeseed, almond, or apricot oil; all are available at health food stores. Just before getting into the tub, add the oil. Watch your footing when getting in and out of the tub, because it will be slippery. Soak for at least 15 minutes, says Zee.

Headache

Tension headaches, which are the most common type, are usually caused by tense muscles in the shoulders, neck, and scalp. When those gnarled-up muscles squeeze the nerves running through them, the irritated nerve endings hammer you with a dull, steady throbbing.

The source of pain in a migraine headache is somewhat different—and more mysterious. People with migraines sometimes experience vomiting, diarrhea, and sensitivity to light and noise, and many doctors believe this combined torture is the result of chemical disturbances in their bodies. Certain foods, alcohol, physical tension, and emotional reactions may release the pain-causing chemicals. The blood vessels in the head constrict temporarily but then swell and become inflamed. While the inflammation decreases the amount of bloodflow to the brain, the swollen vessels press on the nerves.

The Blended Prescription

Note: To learn about cautions and possible side effects of the remedies in this chapter, see page 253.

Since the causes of headaches vary, so do the ways you prevent them—or cure them once they strike. Migraines, in particular, are highly individualized, so if you experience them, work with your doctor to identify the specific causes and treatment. And see a doctor if your non-migraine headaches are getting progressively worse in intensity or frequency; if they are accompanied by confusion, memory loss, dizziness, mood swings, double vision, and coordination problems; or if they followed a fall or blow to the head. But if you are experiencing a garden-variety tension headache—as millions of computer users, school-teachers, and construction workers do—try our blended-medicine experts' three-step nondrug prescription to relieve the headache and prevent it from recurring. If this doesn't work, move on to an over-the-counter painkiller.

Remove yourself from the situation that caused the headache. You cannot make a headache go away if you continue doing what is causing it. So turn off the com-

---

SKILLFUL HEALERS

Acupuncture

Acupuncture can prevent or stop existing headaches, says Alexander Mauskop, M.D., assistant professor of neurology at the State University of New York Health Science Center at Brooklyn, director of the New York Headache Center in New York City, and author of *The Headache Alternative*. Many people believe it helps stimulate the production of endorphins and enkephalins, the body's own pain fighters.

During a course of acupuncture lasting several weeks, you might go once or twice weekly. The acupuncturist inserts thin needles at various points, which might include the sinus area, the webbing between your index finger and thumb, the base of your skull, and a point between your big toe and its neighbor, says Paula G. Maas, D.O., M.D., a homeopathic doctor, chairman of primary care at the Touro University College of Osteopathic Medicine in San Francisco, and author of *The Natural Health Guide to Headache Relief*. The needles might be left in for 20 minutes.

puter, get off the phone, exit the car, get out of the sun, whatever—and find a quiet, comfortable room that you can use in private.

Dim the lights. Bright light is often a headache trigger. Moreover, soft, diffused light is soothing and calming. It is the best environment for releasing tension.

Use isometric exercises to loosen up your shoulder, neck, and scalp muscles. Push one palm against your head above your ear. At the same time, resist the motion by pushing in the opposite direction with your head. Repeat this motion on the opposite side. Next, clasp your hands behind your head to resist as you push your head into them. Then push both hands into your forehead while you resist with your head. Hold each of these exercises for 10 seconds. Try to do this routine 10 times a day.

Other Approaches

For treatment of a headache in progress, take 400 to 600 milligrams of magnesium in cell salt form a day. Cell salt is a type of tablet that you let melt under your tongue and that your body can absorb much faster than a regular pill. Magnesium helps relax the smooth muscles of blood vessels, and if you don't have enough of it, your body may produce a chemical that helps cause inflammation of nerves and headaches. "We estimate that 50 percent of people with migraines are deficient in magnesium," says Alexander Mauskop, M.D., assistant professor of neurology at the State University of New York Health Science Center at Brooklyn, director of the New York Headache Center in New York City, and author of *The Headache Alternative*.

To make sure that you are getting enough magnesium, you can eat foods like nuts, beans, and whole-grain cereals that are high in it. If those foods happen to be among your headache triggers, take 400 to 800 milligrams of magnesium. In addition, take twice as much calcium to aid absorption, says Paula G. Maas, D.O., M.D., a homeopathic doctor, chairman of primary care at the Touro University College of Osteopathic Medicine in San Francisco, and author of *The Natural Health Guide to Headache Relief*. You will also get more absorption if you choose a magnesium supplement that's released slowly into the body, so look for "slow release" on the label, she says.

Limit your caffeine to two servings daily. "Probably the most common cause of frequent headaches is too-high consumption of caffeine," says Dr. Mauskop. What seems contradictory is that caffeine in small amounts can actually help relieve headache pain. In fact, some over-the-counter remedies such as Excedrin contain it. But Dr. Mauskop says to avoid more than two servings of any caffeinated beverages or foods such as coffee, tea, chocolate, cola, and many other sodas.

To find the specific triggers of your pain, keep a headache diary. Many things can trigger a headache, including not only food and alcohol but also unexpected sources such as hair spray and the fumes given off by new carpets. To find the villains, record items like when a headache starts and stops, where the pain was in your head, and what your situation or environment was when the headache started, suggests Dr. Maas. If you also keep a record of various treatments, you can discover your perfect blend of remedies, she says.

Ease a tension headache with a yoga position. Yoga is great for headaches because it helps your body become quiet and relaxed, explains Judith Lasater, Ph.D., a physical therapist in San Francisco and author of *Relax and Renew*. Here's a position that she recommends for both treatment and prevention. You can do this with couch cushions and a thin, rolled-up towel.

HERBAL POWER

Fewer with Feverfew

Feverfew (*Tanacetum parthenium*) is so effective at relieving pain caused by inflammation that it was once nicknamed the headache plant. To relieve pain or prevent future headaches, chew two fresh or freeze-dried feverfew leaves, suggests Alexander Mauskop, M.D., assistant professor of neurology at the State University of New York Health Science Center at Brooklyn, director of the New York Headache Center in New York City, and author of *The Headache Alternative*.

Or you can make a tea with dried feverfew using 2 to 3 tablespoons in one cup of hot water, says Paula G. Maas, D.O., M.D., a homeopathic doctor, chairman of primary care at the Touro University College of Osteopathic Medicine in San Francisco, and author of *The Natural Health Guide to Headache Relief*. Let the tea steep for at least 10 minutes, then strain; add sweeteners to suit your taste. For the best effect, have two cups daily, brewing it fresh every day, she says.

- Line up cushions lengthwise to create a floor mat the length of your body.
- Lie on your back so your head and shoulders are lightly touching the floor with the rest of your body on the cushions. This will stretch the muscles at the back and sides of your neck.
- Place the rolled-up towel under the base of your neck and the top of your shoulders so your head is supported comfortably.
- If you feel uncomfortable, bend your knees, placing one foot on either side of the cushions or both on top.

• Once you are comfortable in this position, with your jaw and tongue completely relaxed, focus on releasing the tension from your neck and head. Breathe soft and comfortably long breaths. Hold the position for 5 to 15 minutes.

This yoga position can also be done with folded-up blankets under you or with an exercise mat if you have one.

Wrap your head with a 6- to 8-inch-wide elastic bandage. You will increase the benefit of any yoga position done to relieve a headache if you wrap your head with an elastic bandage, Dr. Lasater says. Starting at the base of your skull, wrap the bandage around your head until it covers your eyes. Tuck in the end to hold it in place. The bandage puts a comfortable amount of pressure on your temples, sinuses, and forehead while blocking out light.

To help prevent headaches, take 40 milligrams of ginkgo three times a day. Ginkgo (*Ginkgo biloba*) helps increase bloodflow to the brain, says Dr. Mauskop, and it also helps prevent your blood from forming dangerous clots. Be patient, though. "It might take up to 6 weeks before a person stops getting headaches," he notes.

Every hour or so, roll your shoulders. Relaxing tense shoulders just might help you get rid of headaches for good, especially the tension variety. The trapezoid muscles—the ones that lift your shoulders when you are tense—are "wired" to transmit pain signals to the brain. But you can ease the muscles and prevent the pain if you roll your shoulders in a giant circle. Keeping your arms at your sides, roll your shoulders in a clockwise motion for a few minutes. Then reverse and roll them in a counterclockwise motion, suggests Dr. Mauskop.

Mix up some ginger tea. At the first sign of a headache, mix ⅓ teaspoon of powdered or grated fresh ginger (*Zin-*

giber officinale) into one cup of hot water. Let cool, strain, and drink, says Dr. Maas. Ginger quiets the inflamed blood vessels in your head, slows the release of the body's pain-sensitizing chemicals, and improves circulation.

Apply a solution of peppermint (*Mentha piperita*) essential oil and alcohol to your shoulders, neck, and face. According to published research, this solution cools your skin, and the peppermint scent helps relieve stress, says Kurt Schnaubelt, Ph.D., scientific director of the Pacific Institute of Aromatherapy in San Rafael, California. To make the solution, mix 2 tablespoons of peppermint oil with 1 cup of rubbing alcohol. Apply the solution liberally, but be careful not to get it in your eyes or mouth, he adds.

Take aspirin with acetaminophen, but not with ibuprofen. Over-the-counter headache drugs help to stop inflammation and block pain-producing chemicals, says Dr. Maas. If you take a painkiller that contains aspirin and don't get the result you want in 20 to 60 minutes, you can immediately take a drug that contains acetaminophen, such as Tylenol, Dr. Maas says. But to avoid side effects, don't take aspirin with ibuprofen since they have the same active ingredients, she explains.

Heartburn

When all's going well, the food you eat moves smoothly toward your stomach. The problem arises—literally—when there is a welling up from down below, and stomach acid backs up.

This only happens when an important little trapdoor, called the lower esophageal sphincter, malfunctions. This muscle, located at the junction of the esophagus and stomach, keeps the stomach's highly acidic hydrochloric acid from seeping upward. When the sphincter weakens or relaxes inappropriately, a regurgitation of stomach acid rushes up your esophagus. You experience a burning sensation in your upper chest area as sensitive tissues get irritated by the acid. Heartburn usually occurs after large meals and can last a few minutes to several hours.

The Blended Prescription

Note: To learn about cautions and possible side effects of the remedies in this chapter, see page 253.

Severe heartburn can sometimes mimic the symptoms of a heart attack, stomach ulcer, or hiatal hernia. See your doctor if your heartburn is severe or prolonged or if it persists for 15 minutes after taking an antacid.

Easy remedies to calm mild to moderate heartburn are within your reach. You also may avoid this condition by knowing which foods are more likely to give you heartburn. Here are the seven best conventional and natural solutions recommended by our blended-medicine experts.

When heartburn hits, lie down on your left side. This position keeps the stomach below the esophagus.

Drink a large glass of lukewarm water. Doing this will help dilute the acid and flush it through the digestive system.

Take an over-the-counter antacid to neutralize your overflowing gastric juices. Antacids are among the most commonly used drugs in America, so there are dozens to choose from: Gaviscon, Maalox, Mylanta, Tums, Rolaids, and more. They differ primarily in what mineral they use to neutralize the acid (aluminum, calcium, magnesium, and sodium are most common). Try different brands until you find the one that works best for you.

Drink 2 ounces of aloe vera juice as needed. The juice will help soothe the irritated esophagus and stomach lining.

Chew two deglycyrrhizinated licorice wafers every 2 to 3 hours. Licorice root (*Glycyrrhiza glabra*) is a natural antispasmodic that also reduces stomach acid production.

Have a cup or two of herbal tea. Try tea made with one of the following herbs: slippery elm (*Ulmus rubra*), marshmallow (*Althaea officinalis*), ginger (*Zingiber officinale*), or plantain (*Plantago*, various species). All these teas have stomach-soothing properties.

For heartburn that comes after eating rich food, take the homeopathic remedy Nux vomica 6C. If the heartburn comes after little food, take Lycopodium 6C. Take Carbo vegetabilis 6C if you have burning in your stomach with an acid taste in your mouth. The dosage is two pellets every 15 minutes for four doses, and then two pellets every hour until the symptoms subside.

Other Approaches

To avoid heartburn, don't eat peppermint or chocolate before going to sleep. These foods relax the lower esophageal sphincter so that stomach acid vapors can flood back up when you lie down to sleep, warns Dale Anderson, M.D., clinical assistant professor at the University of Minnesota Medical School in Minneapolis. "That's why you should never eat those chocolate mints placed on your hotel pillow at night," he says. "Save them for the next day."

Sidestep heartburn-producing foods. Coffee, alcohol, milk, spicy foods, orange juice, and fried foods are known to aggravate your digestive system, says Mark Stengler, N.D., a naturopathic physician in Carlsbad, California, and author of *The Natural Physician*. These foods contain substances that can provoke an excess production of stomach acid and weaken your lower esophageal sphincter muscle.

Eat five to six small meals daily. Instead of consuming three large meals a day, try eating five or six smaller meals to give your digestive system the time and strength to properly break down your foods, suggests Dr. Anderson.

Combat mild heartburn by chewing gum. Gum chewing stimulates saliva, which can soothe your irritated esophagus, says Jorge Herrera, M.D., professor of medicine in the division of gastroenterology at the University of South Alabama College of Medicine in Mobile.

Dine on a hearty, heartburn-free salad. Certain foods are very mild to your digestive tract and can stimulate your liver, gallbladder, and stomach to digest more efficiently, Dr. Stengler says. He recommends munching on a salad containing these anti-heartburn ingredients: lettuce, almonds, dandelion, garlic, chicory, mustard, olives, and walnuts.

Prepare for a night of beer and pizza by taking Pepcid AC, Zantac, or Tagamet in advance. These over-the-counter histamine receptor blockers (H_2 blockers) take about 30 minutes to an hour to enter your bloodstream and prevent your stomach from secreting hydrochloric acid back up the esophagus, says Dr. Herrera. "They work very well as heartburn preventives."

Hemorrhoids

Little veins in and around your rectum and anus normally expand during a bowel movement and shrink back to their normal shape after the stools exit. The expansion-contraction sequence works in harmony until undue pressure is placed on these veins, which can happen if you spend a lot of time sitting or put strain on that area when you lift heavy objects. A saclike protrusion, called a

HERBAL POWER

A Broom and a Nut

Shrink swollen hemorrhoidal tissue with a pair of herbs, advises Mark Stengler, N.D., a naturopathic physician in Carlsbad, California, and author of *The Natural Physician*. His favorites are butcher's broom (*Ruscus aculeatus*) and horse chestnut (*Aesculus hippocastanum*). The dosage for butcher's broom is one 150-milligram capsule or 30 drops of the tincture three times daily. For horse chestnut, it is one 50-milligram capsule or 30 drops of the tincture three times daily. Take these herbs until the tissues return to their normal shape.

"When you take these herbs, blood vessel inflammation decreases, and tissues tighten," explains Dr. Stengler.

hemorrhoid, can form in the area of strain, and sometimes the tiny blood vessels rupture and bleed.

You won't feel hemorrhoids that are inside your anus, because the internal membranes lack pain-sensitive nerve fibers. Then there are external hemorrhoids, which hurt because they push out like a water-filled balloon to form a swollen lump outside your anus.

The Blended Prescription

Note: To learn about cautions and possible side effects of the remedies in this chapter, see page 253.

You should see a doctor if you experience persistent pain, bleeding in the rectum, or blood in your stool that lasts for more than a few days. That bleeding could be a symptom of colorectal cancer. If your hemorrhoids don't require medical attention, drugstore solutions may be the quickest and best way to reduce the swelling and irritation. Here is a five-step prescription from our blended-medicine experts.

When hemorrhoids are uncomfortable and aggravating, take sitz baths. Fill a tub with 4 inches of water that is as hot as you can tolerate, add ½ cup of witch hazel, and place a thick, folded terry-cloth towel in the tub. Ease yourself in and sit on the towel with cheeks spread for 10 to 15 minutes, three times a day.

Wipe with a witch hazel compress instead of dry toilet paper. Witch hazel is an astringent that soothes soreness and itchiness. Buy pretreated compresses like Tucks Pads, or moisten toilet paper with witch hazel.

Take acetaminophen or aspirin, following the label instructions. These over-the-counter medications help ease pain.

Apply an over-the-counter 1 percent hydrocortisone cream, according to the package directions. This medication helps soothe the itching.

Use drugstore hemorrhoidal suppositories (such as Preparation H) or a hemorrhoidal ointment (such as Anusol). These remedies ease the discomfort.

Other Approaches

Perform aerobic exercise three times a week for 20 to 30 minutes each time. Choose an aerobic exercise that you enjoy, and make it a part of your life, says Mark Stengler, N.D., a naturopathic physician in Carlsbad, California, and author of *The Natural Physician*. Brisk walking, cycling, ballroom dancing, and especially swimming are all good aerobic activities. The goal is to regularly increase circulation to your pelvic area and reduce venous congestion to keep muscle tone and maintain the quality of your veins, he notes.

Drink 4 ounces of dark berry juice mixed with 4 ounces of apple juice. Cherries, blackberries, and blueberries all contain bioflavonoids, which strengthen the walls of veins and capillaries, says Andrew T. Weil, M.D., clinical professor of internal medicine and director of the integrative medicine program at the University of Arizona College of Medicine in Tucson and author of *Spontaneous Healing*. So these juices have a healing effect while also promoting regularity.

Eat 40 grams of fiber every day. Foods high in fiber, especially fruits, vegetables, and whole grains, provide roughage to help digested food move smoothly through the intestines and colon, says Dr. Stengler. He says that eating 40 grams of fiber a day helps prevent straining of your pelvic muscles and reduces congestion of the rectal veins, the causes of hemorrhoids.

See your doctor to have hemorrhoids removed. Sometimes a minor outpatient procedure is necessary to remove persistent internal hemorrhoids. Your doctor may recommend what is called a rubber band ligation, says Lester Rosen, M.D., a colon-rectal surgeon in group practice in Allentown, Pennsylvania. One or two tiny rubber bands are placed around the base of the hemorrhoid to cut off circulation. "It is usually done painlessly, with no need for anesthetic," he says. "It is a minor, safe procedure." Within 10 days, the appendage falls off and the area heals, he adds.

High Blood Pressure

In a healthy person, blood flows smoothly and efficiently through clean, wide arteries, powered along by a strong heart. Pressure is low. But with neglect, so many things can go wrong. Cholesterol-clogged and hardened arteries are a major cause for blood pressure to rise. Excessive salt in the diet draws fluid into the blood, increasing volume in the arterial space. Being overweight can increase pressure, merely by forcing the heart to beat harder to get blood to all those fleshy hills and valleys. Race and genetics can contribute as well.

The problem with high blood pressure is that you can't feel it. Silently, it can cause your heart to enlarge. It can scar and harden your arteries. And it may contribute to heart attacks, strokes, kidney failure, and eye damage. As many as 50 million Americans have been diagnosed with high blood pressure, says the American Heart Association.

The Blended Prescription

Note: To learn about cautions and possible side effects of the remedies in this chapter, see page 253.

There are many tried-and-true methods to lower blood pressure, which work even better blended. Many are lifestyle changes of a high magnitude. We'll just touch on them, even though they are the most important. In addition, many supplements and herbs can help reduce the pressure. Here is a 10-part prescription from our team of blended-medicine experts to lower blood pressure.

Improve the quality of your diet. Start by reducing or eliminating processed foods, salted foods, sugary foods, and caffeine. Likewise, cut back on meat products. The closer your diet is to vegetarian, the better it is for your blood pressure.

Take care of the other big-picture health challenges. Lose excess weight, stop smoking, and exercise regularly. Each of these will have a significant effect on your blood pressure. Indeed, each can add years—high-quality years—to your life.

Reduce unnecessary stress in your life, and learn to cope better with the necessary stresses. This is one area in which professional help makes sense. Seriously consider getting professional training in any of the popular stress-relief methods: meditation, tai chi, and yoga.

Take 350 milligrams of magnesium every day. Magnesium is a particularly heart-healthy mineral that helps arteries stay clean and open. Studies confirm that it also helps control high blood pressure. Try getting more magnesium from foods, advises Jerry Hickey, R.Ph., chairman of the Society of Natural Pharmacy and cohost of the radio show *Healthline*. Good sources include green leafy vegetables, whole grains, brown rice, legumes, and nuts. But with your doctor's consent, magnesium supplements—sometimes in conjunction with calcium supplements—may be appropriate for battling high blood pressure.

Take an antioxidant combination each day. Find a supplement that includes beta-carotene, vitamins C and E, and selenium. Antioxidants eradicate artery-damaging molecules called free radicals.

If you have given up smoking, beta-carotene and selenium, in particular, are important supplements to take. They can help repair cells in the lining of lungs damaged by smoking, according to David Field, N.D., a naturopathic physician and licensed acupuncturist in Santa Rosa, California.

Use two heart-friendly amino-acid supplements—carnitine and arginine. Take 500 milligrams of each three times a day.

Twice a day, take 50 milligrams of coenzyme Q_{10}. It's a supplement that many believe is beneficial for the heart.

Take 250 milligrams of hawthorn (*Crataegus laevigata*) in standardized extract form three times a day. Hawthorn extracts, taken from the berries of the English hawthorn tree, contain chemicals called polyphenols that are particularly good for your heart in two ways. First, they dilate blood vessels, particularly coronary arteries, helping to reduce blood pressure. Second, they help improve heart function when taken over a long period.

Eat lots of fresh garlic, or take 320 milligrams of garlic extract once or twice a day. Perhaps the world's most popular medicinal food, garlic appears to lower cholesterol in the bloodstream and reduces blood pressure. Just ½ ounce per week (about a clove a day) can reduce high blood pressure.

Take prescription drugs as directed by your physician. By definition, they require your doctor's consent and are powerful. Always take them exactly as directed, and quickly report side effects so that your doctor can change your prescription if necessary. Most important, make the lifestyle changes you need to control high blood pressure through more-natural methods. Your goal is to get off blood pressure medications quickly and permanently.

High Cholesterol

Your heart is an engine, a fist-size machine of chambers and valves that motor your body through its daily activities. In synchronized rhythm, a circuitry of pipes works to deliver the rich fuel of blood throughout your body. But when a fatty substance called low-density lipoprotein (LDL) cholesterol builds up as plaque along the walls of your arteries, the pipes get clogged. The blood no longer sweeps through but instead squeezes through, depriving your heart of its full amount of fuel and disrupting the delicate harmony of circulation.

This is when your body enlists the help of high-density

lipoprotein (HDL) cholesterol to vacuum the blood clean of the impurities left by LDL and ferry it back to the liver. The liver then breaks down the debris and eliminates it from your body. If a blood test reveals that you are housing too much LDL and not enough HDL to keep it from accumulating, you run the risk of heart disease.

The Blended Prescription

Note: To learn about cautions and possible side effects of the remedies in this chapter, see page 253.

Your cholesterol levels are directly affected by the amount of animal fat in your diet. A desirable number for total cholesterol is below 200. If your cholesterol is only slightly elevated (between 200 and 239) and heart disease doesn't run in your family, limit your calories from fat to 20 to 30 percent of your total calories, says Lee Lipsenthal, M.D., medical director of the Preventive Medicine Research Institute in Sausalito, California. If your level is high (above 239) or if heart disease runs in your family, stick with a diet recommended by your doctor, who might also recommend cholesterol-lowering drugs.

If your cholesterol levels are elevated (even slightly) or you have a high genetic risk for heart disease, you should get a cholesterol blood test every 6 months until your cholesterol normalizes. Have your cholesterol levels checked yearly if they're in the normal range. Beyond smart nutrition, here are eight steps that you can take together to get your cholesterol levels down as fast as possible, as prescribed by our blended-medicine experts.

Exercise three or four times a week. Regular activity that raises your heart rate reduces your LDL levels and increases your HDL levels. It also builds up your heart so that it can pump more blood with less effort. Consistency is key, so weekend warriors take note: A 4-hour bike ride on Saturday doesn't mean that you can be a couch potato the rest of the week. Your heart will benefit more if you divide your exercise time into 30- to 40-minute workouts

---

HERBAL POWER

A Field of Medicine

With your doctor's approval, try adding these herbal remedies to your personal cholesterol-reduction program.

Lime tree flower (Tilia platyphyllos) helps remove plaque buildup in the arteries and guards against cholesterol deposits, says Cheri Annette Wagner, a member of the National Institute of Medical Herbalists and an herbalist at Equipoise Center of America in Rochester, New York. Drink the tea three times a day after every meal, she suggests.

Globe artichoke (Cynara scolymus) helps escort cholesterol from the body and stimulates the liver, aiding in the digestion of fats. Take 500 milligrams a day in capsule form until your levels normalize, Wagner advises.

Guar gum (Cyamopsis tetragonolobus) is considered by herbalists to be good at lowering blood-fat levels. Take 1 teaspoon a day in dry, granular form, and accompany it with at least 8 ounces of water.

Guggul (Commiphora mukul) is extremely effective in improving high-density lipoprotein levels and lowering total cholesterol levels, says Chris Meletis, N.D., professor of natural pharmacology and nutrition, dean of clinical education, and chief medical officer at the National College of Naturopathic Medicine in Portland, Oregon. Take 500 milligrams in capsule form two or three times a day until your cholesterol normalizes.

throughout the week. It is better to do some type of activity each day rather than lots in 1 or 2 days.

Add fiber-rich foods to your diet. Soluble fiber can reduce your total cholesterol level by up to 10 percent. Fiber, found in foods like oat bran and legumes, acts like a digestive mop, sopping up LDL cholesterol and other digestive litter and swiftly showing them the door. Fiber also has the added benefit of helping you control your weight by making you feel full.

Drink six to eight glasses of water a day. If you are regularly constipated, you will have a buildup of cholesterol in your stool waiting to be eliminated. While it's in a holding pattern, it could get reabsorbed in the bloodstream, says Chris Meletis, N.D., professor of natural pharmacology and nutrition, dean of clinical education, and chief medical officer at the National College of Naturopathic Medicine in Portland, Oregon. Water helps prevent constipation and keeps things flowing.

Take 1½ teaspoons of flaxseed (*Linum usitatissimum*) oil every day. The oil from these shiny, hard seeds is a rich source of omega-3 fatty acids, a heart-healthy fat that lowers LDL levels and helps prevent blood clots. One-and-a-half tablespoons of the ground seed is just as omega-rich as the oil, and it also contains fiber. The ground seed can be added to food like cereal and yogurt every day.

Take vitamins C and E and beta-carotene every day. Their antioxidant properties help your body metabolize cholesterol and stop free-radical formation, which is damaging to the artery walls. Take 2,000 milligrams of vitamin C, 400 international units (IU) of vitamin E, and 50,000 IU of beta-carotene every day.

Use olive oil when cooking. It is a monounsaturated oil that can help reduce cholesterol levels in the bloodstream and is a particularly heart-healthy food.

Stop smoking and cut back on alcohol and caffeine. Tobacco smoke suppresses HDL cholesterol and can damage your heart and arteries. And excessive amounts of alcohol or caffeine—more than two glasses or cups per day—can increase the risk of cholesterol-related heart disease.

See your doctor about niacin supplements. Otherwise known as vitamin B_3, niacin is particularly good at lowering triglyceride and LDL levels and raising HDL levels. Although it is completely safe in the small doses that occur in foods or multivitamins, when taken in supplement form, niacin is more like a drug, with many possible side effects. So be sure to take it under a doctor's supervision. The prescribed amount likely would be far above the recommended Daily Value of 20 milligrams. There are two types of niacin supplements: nicotinic acid and nicotinamide. Be sure that you get nicotinic acid since nicotinamide has been found not to lower cholesterol. Ask your doctor to recommend a variety that won't cause flushing.

Other Approaches

Get hooked on fish once a day. Like flaxseed oil, fish—especially deep-cold-water fish—is a powerhouse of heart-healthy omega-3 fatty acids, notes Dr. Meletis. Halibut, cod, and red snapper are good choices, he says.

Avoid iron. Since iron is an oxidant, it can actually enhance plaque formation, says Dr. Lipsenthal. Unless you have anemia or are menstruating heavily, avoid supplements that contain iron, he says.

Balance your cholesterol levels with one to three cloves of garlic a day. Garlic is an approved remedy for high cholesterol in Europe, according to James A. Duke, Ph.D., a botanical consultant, a former ethnobotanist with the U.S. Department of Agriculture who specializes in medicinal plants, and author of *The Green Pharmacy*.

Raw garlic is best. "When you cook garlic, you lose the treasure of it," says Cheri Annette Wagner, a member of the National Institute of Medical Herbalists and an herbalist at Equipoise Center of America in Rochester, New York. If social fears prevent you from noshing on this odoriferous herb, Wagner suggests taking two odorless garlic supplements three times a day. Look for a brand that says it is standardized to at least 1.3 percent allicin, she adds.

Eat half an onion a day. This amount has been shown to lower total cholesterol levels by 10 to 15 percent, says Dr. Duke. Onion is milder than garlic and may be preferable if you can't tolerate its pungent cousin, suggests Wagner. Again, raw gives you the most benefits.

Learn meditation. It is perhaps the most relaxing form of stress management there is, notes Dr. Lipsenthal. Stress drives up your production of adrenaline, which increases triglyceride levels, another fatty acid linked to heart disease. By raising your awareness of breathing, meditation redirects your thoughts into a world that is calm and tranquil. Working with a teacher is important because most people can't go from a state of business to sitting quietly without some coaching, he says.

Practice yoga. Focusing on the gentle rhythm of breathing and the fluid movements of muscles has a calming effect much like meditation, according to Dr. Lipsenthal. Any yoga position has a relaxing outcome, he says. For help in locating a yoga teacher in your area, contact the American Yoga Foundation at 40 School House Road, Bovina Center, NY 13740.

Find a hobby. If meditation or yoga isn't your style, find a hobby that enables you to "lose yourself," suggests Dr. Lipsenthal. A well-suited hobby, whether it is fly-fishing or needlepoint, transports you to a world where time slips away without notice and daily woes don't exist, he says.

If high cholesterol is a serious concern for you, talk with your doctor about whether a prescription drug is appropriate. Your doctor will profile you and your risk factors (age, LDL level, family heart history, smoking, diabetes, and so on) to see what is an appropriate cholesterol level for you. A prescription drug may be recommended if lifestyle changes won't be enough to solve the problem, says Robert DiBianco, M.D., associate clinical professor of medicine at Georgetown University School of Medicine in Washington, D.C., and cardiologist and director of cardiology research at Washington Adventist Hospital in Takoma Park, Maryland. If you qualify for treatment, there are several types of medications that can be used.

Statins. They decrease cholesterol production by the liver and cause the liver to remove LDL cholesterol from the blood. They also raise HDL levels. Statins are the most commonly prescribed drug for reducing coronary risks, says Dr. DiBianco.

Nicotinic acid. Commonly known as niacin, this vitamin lowers LDL and triglyceride levels and raises HDL levels.

Bile acid binding agents. They bind bile acids in the intestine, which forces the liver to pull more cholesterol from the blood to form more bile acids. As a result, your cholesterol levels fall. Bile acid binding agents are among the oldest medications used, says Dr. DiBianco.

Hives

Fish, insect venom, milk, penicillin, and nuts are just some of the substances that can cause the allergic reaction known as hives, but there are many other potential causes as well. Whatever the cause, the reaction in your body triggers the release of the powerful chemicals called histamines that are only partially counteracted by anti-inflammatory chemicals from the adrenal gland. Notorious for their role in hay fever and colds, histamines make the blood vessels dilate and leak fluid into the surrounding tissue, which in turn causes redness, pain, and inflammation. Hives, the end result of this reaction, are itchy, burning welts that typically appear on the skin.

The Blended Prescription

Note: To learn about cautions and possible side effects of the remedies in this chapter, see page 253.

If you have hives that last longer than 24 hours or hives that leave a bruise after they go away, check with your doctor. You should go to the emergency room if you have hives around your eyes or mouth or if you have difficulty breathing. But for a case of ordinary hives, you have plenty of time for a more measured response with these seven tactics from our blended-medicine experts.

Get an over-the-counter antihistamine (such as Benadryl) from the drugstore. Take 25 to 50 milligrams three times a day as needed, paying attention to the cautions on the label. (Drivers' alert: It makes you drowsy.) In many cases, this remedy may be the only one you will need to find relief.

Take 1,000 milligrams of vitamin C three times a day. Vitamin C is known for its antihistamine action, which may help to reduce hives.

Three times a day, take 300 to 500 milligrams of quercetin or any mixture of bioflavonoids. Bioflavonoids, which are sold as nutritional supplements, give many fruits and vegetables their hue. Scientists have identified more than 800 bioflavonoids (quercetin is one of the most

HERBAL POWER

A Nettle That Works like Magic

Stinging nettle (*Urtica dioica*) helps soothe hives, says Shiva Barton, N.D., a licensed acupuncturist and lead naturopathic physician at the Wellspace Health Center in Cambridge, Massachusetts. Although the plant has histamines that can make your skin swell, it also has properties that can help your hives disappear. Take 450 to 550 milligrams every 2 to 4 hours as needed to relieve symptoms, he says.

common), and some believe they are effective at battling allergic reactions.

Supplement your nutrients with three daily doses of 500 milligrams of pantothenic acid. It's known to stimulate the adrenal gland to produce cortisol, your body's own anti-inflammatory.

Have three 1,000-milligram fish-oil capsules every day. The oil has anti-inflammatory properties that can help reduce hives. Continue this therapy until the hives disappear.

Use a homeopathic dose of Apis mellifica 6C. Take two pellets every 15 minutes for four doses. As the hives begin to go away, take two pellets every hour for four doses.

Add a cup of an oatmeal powder (such as Aveeno) to a tub of cool water. The oatmeal acts as a soothing agent against itching and irritation. Soak in it for 20 to 30 minutes.

Other Approaches

Rub your foot for a minute or two. There is an acupressure point on the bottom exact middle of your foot (right in the arch) that proponents believe stimulates the adrenal gland to send out anti-inflammatory chemicals to reduce the swelling of hives. If you press and rub firmly on that point, your hives should begin going down within 20 minutes, says Shiva Barton, N.D., a licensed acupuncturist and lead naturopathic physician at the Wellspace Health Center in Cambridge, Massachusetts.

Avoid the triggers. Try to recall what you ate or what came in contact with your skin just before each outbreak of hives, says Dr. Barton. If you suspect a food allergy but can't figure out exactly which food doesn't like you, ask your doctor for an IgG blood test. This test can tell which foods—or food groups—may be causing the allergic reaction.

Arm yourself with protection. Serious symptoms can hit fast if you have a violent allergic reaction. Hives inside your mouth, for example, could narrow your airways, putting you at risk for suffocation.

If you know you are allergy prone and you've had hives before, ask your doctor if you should be carrying a kit that contains epinephrine injections to help handle life-threatening hives, says Dee Anna Glaser, M.D., assistant professor of dermatology at St. Louis University School of Medicine in Missouri. Epinephrine is a prescription anti-inflammatory drug, and a physician can show you how to administer it yourself so that you will be prepared if you ever need to use it fast.

Indigestion

Proper digestion begins with proper chewing. If you take big bites and swallow quickly, your stomach can't store all the arriving food and liquids. Moreover, your stomach doesn't have enough digestive secretions and enzymes to thoroughly wash the food when it arrives.

When it is pressured into high-speed processing, your stomach ends up shipping partially digested or undigested food into your small intestine and colon. There, the undigested portions ferment, producing hydrogen and carbon dioxide. As a result, you are likely to feel gassy, bloated, and cramped—all symptoms of indigestion.

Stress and worry can add to your digestive woes. So can certain foods and beverages that are irritating to the digestive tract, including alcohol, vinegar, caffeine, greasy or spicy foods, and gum with sorbitol.

The Blended Prescription

Note: To learn about cautions and possible side effects of the remedies in this chapter, see page 253.

If your indigestion is accompanied by nausea, vomiting, fever, or bloody stools, see your doctor to rule out a more serious condition, such as an ulcer. Otherwise, the obvious first step is to eat slowly and chew thoroughly. And when indigestion hits, use this six-step prescription for relief, as prescribed by our blended-medicine experts.

Stop smoking, and don't consume fatty fried foods, caffeine, alcohol, and refined sugars. All slow down your digestive process and increase your chance for indigestion, cautions Mark Stengler, N.D., a naturopathic physician in Carlsbad, California, and author of *The Natural Physician*.

Take some Pepto-Bismol, following the package instructions. Yes, this old standby of digestive medicine remains one of the best. That said, most over-the-counter indigestion medicines work well. Consider Gaviscon for heartburn, Gas-X for gas, and Mylanta or Maalox for burning sensations in the stomach. Whatever you do,

HERBAL POWER

Cayenne for Digestion

High in vitamins A and C, cayenne pepper (*Capsicum,* various species) is a powerful tonic that stimulates the heart, promotes circulation, improves digestion, and boosts energy. It is believed that this spicy pepper stimulates bloodflow and increases nutrients to your stomach lining, says David J. Nickel, O.M.D., a doctor of Oriental medicine and licensed acupuncturist in Santa Monica, California. You can sprinkle cayenne pepper on your favorite food or swallow it in capsule form. Or you can stir 1 teaspoon into a cup of boiling water, steep for 10 minutes, and drink it as an herbal tea.

don't take any medicine with aspirin in it since aspirin can damage your stomach lining.

Make a cup of herbal tea after eating or at the onset of indigestion to soothe your beastly stomach. The best choices include chamomile (*Matricaria recutita*), peppermint (*Mentha piperita*), and ginger (*Zingiber officinale*).

Take two or three capsules (500 to 750 milligrams total) of activated charcoal at the first signs of indigestion. "Charcoal is excellent for indigestion, especially when you have gas and bloating," says David J. Nickel, O.M.D., a doctor of Oriental medicine and licensed acupuncturist in Santa Monica, California. For faster results, open the capsules in a half-glass of warm water, stir to dissolve, and drink. Don't worry if your stool is blackened for a day or two while you take activated charcoal. In most cases, the charcoal absorbs unwanted gas and provides significant relief within 15 to 30 minutes.

If indigestion is frequent, see if taking digestive enzymes with your meals helps. These supplements are available at any health food store. One capsule of digestive enzymes is usually swallowed at the beginning of a meal, but follow the package instructions carefully.

Apply acupressure to the webbed area between your thumb and index finger. This acupressure point relaxes your entire digestive system, says Dr. Nickel. To apply pressure, use the thumb and forefinger of one hand to pinch the webbed area of the opposite hand. As you squeeze, slide around the finger that is on the outside of the webbed area to probe for the acupressure point. You'll know when you find it because your squeezing will create an aching or hurting sensation in the web. That's one of

---

SKILLFUL HEALERS

Aromatherapy

Consider visiting a licensed aromatherapist if indigestion is a repeated problem for you. Essential oils can stimulate or sedate your digestive system, says David J. Nickel, O.M.D., a doctor of Oriental medicine and licensed acupuncturist in Santa Monica, California. An aroma expert can help you select the right scents to reactivate your digestive juices, he adds.

For indigestion, Victoria Edwards, an aromatherapist and owner of Leydet Aromatics in Fair Oaks, California, says she often applies on a person's stomach one or two drops each of peppermint (*Mentha piperita*), rosemary (*Rosmarinus officinalis*), and lavender (*Lavandula angustifolia*) essential oils mixed with a dab of olive oil. She gently blends these oils into the skin, which releases their aromas at the same time.

the acupressure points that connect with your digestive and elimination systems, according to Dr. Nickel. As you press, exhale through your mouth and inhale through your nose. Maintain the pressure for about 2 to 3 minutes, or until you feel a "good" hurt.

Other Approaches

Swallow two 500-milligram capsules of garlic three times a day with meals. Garlic aids in digestion and kills bad bacteria, says Dr. Nickel. It also assists the mineral zinc, which is essential in helping pancreatic enzymes break down protein. "Garlic is extremely high in sulfur, and sulfur is a major binder that makes zinc work effectively for digestion," he explains.

Gargle with ½ teaspoon of natural sea salt stirred in a glass of warm water. Sea salt contains mainly sodium and chloride, which help stimulate your hydrochloric acid in digesting food, says Dr. Nickel. You can also salt your food for the same benefits.

Avoid gum chewing after you eat a big meal. Each time you chew gum, you swallow air. It's no wonder that you feel bloated, gassy, and uncomfortable, says Malcolm Robinson, M.D., a gastroenterologist at the University of Oklahoma Health Sciences Center in Oklahoma City.

Don't exercise vigorously right after eating a meal. "Around mealtime, about 35 percent of your body's energy is used in digestion," says Dr. Nickel. "The less energy you have for digestion, the longer it takes to break down your food." If you exercise right after eating, you shift your body's circulation away from your digestive system and toward your muscles, inhibiting digestion. It is best to wait at least an hour after eating before you exercise, he recommends.

Take the homeopathic remedy Carbo vegetabilis 30C two or three times a day. Homeopathic doctors are likely to recommend this cure when you feel heaviness in your stomach accompanied by sour-tasting burps, flatulence, and a burning sensation in your chest, says Jennifer Jacobs, M.D., a homeopathic physician, assistant clinical professor of epidemiology at the University of Washington in Edmonds, and coauthor of *Healing with Homeopathy*. If you don't see improvement after 2 days, discontinue using the remedy. If your indigestion is from rich and fatty foods, try another homeopathic remedy: Pulsatilla 6C.

Insect Stings and Bites

Your body reacts instantly to a bee's venom or a mosquito's salivary secretions. Why? Both are foreign proteins that your body doesn't recognize. So you develop an allergic response of varying severity, with in-rushing histamines causing the familiar redness around the sting.

The Blended Prescription

Note: To learn about cautions and possible side effects of the remedies in this chapter, see page 253.

See a medical doctor immediately if you experience difficulty breathing, dizziness, or severe itching or if your lips, eyes, and tongue start to swell after a bee sting. You could be having a serious allergic reaction.

If you are not allergic and you have been attacked by insects, use soap and water to clean the puncture area. If you have been stung by a bee, remove the stinger by scraping the edge of a credit card over the area. Hold the card at a 90-degree angle and flick the stinger off. After that, you can use this full-circle approach recommended by our blended-medicine experts.

To relieve the itch and pain, apply one of the following, depending on availability and what works best for you. Try ice, calamine lotion, baking soda paste (baking soda mixed with a few drops of water), one drop of essential oil of lavender (*Lavandula officinalis*), or nonprescription 1 percent hydrocortisone cream.

Treat it homeopathically with two pellets of Ledum 6C or Apis mellifica 6C taken every 15 minutes for four doses, then two pellets every hour for four doses on the first day. After that, take two pellets four times a day until your symptoms resolve.

Swallow 1,000 milligrams of vitamin C once a day and 500 milligrams of quercetin three times a day to treat bee stings. Vitamin C and quercetin (a bioflavonoid) may help reduce inflammation, says Mark Michaud, M.D., a family physician with American WholeHealth Centers in Chicago.

Insomnia

To get its well-deserved rest, your body relies on the hormone melatonin, which is secreted by a gland in your brain. If all goes smoothly, the melatonin level in your system rises dramatically before bedtime, and every fiber of your body starts prompting you to get some rest. By the time you flop into bed, your mind and body are responding to the melatonin-induced signals that tell you to relax and drift off.

When you have insomnia, something goes awry. Either there is not enough melatonin in your system or other signals are working overtime to keep you awake or even waken you in the middle of the night. Among the sleep robbers are emotional states like depression and anxiety as well as certain foods and drinks, particularly those that contain alcohol or caffeine. Physical pain can override the power of melatonin, and so can some medications that have a stimulating effect on your body.

The Blended Prescription

Note: To learn about cautions and possible side effects of the remedies in this chapter, see page 253.

See an M.D. if you have insomnia for more than a month, need to use medications to fall asleep, or are so sleep-deprived that you have trouble functioning normally during the day.

To combat insomnia on your own, you must boost your level of melatonin when you most need it or implement some relaxation techniques that allow your natural supply of this hormone to work effectively. Besides melatonin supplements, many other remedies can help, but you need to take them on a rotational basis: A single supplement can lose its effectiveness if you use it too frequently. So the first of our six steps offers you a wide range of supplement choices. Here's what our blended-medicine panel recommends.

Try any of the following natural supplements ½ hour to 1 hour before bedtime to help you sleep. All of these supplements have a soothing effect and help to relax and calm you.

Melatonin: 1 to 3 milligrams

Valerian (Valeriana officinalis): 150 to 300 milligrams

Passionflower (Passiflora incarnata): 300 to 450 milligrams

Kava kava (Piper methysticum): 70 to 140 milligrams

Hydroxytryptophan (S-HTP, an amino acid): 100 to 300 milligrams

HERBAL POWER

Sleep with Valerian

The herb valerian (*Valeriana officinalis*) helps you sleep by quieting your central nervous system, says Brigitte Mars, a professional member of the American Herbalists Guild and a clinical herbalist with UniTea Herbs in Boulder, Colorado. It works like a mild sedative. Take one capsule of valerian root extract 30 to 45 minutes before going to bed, she suggests. Because capsules come in various potencies, Mars suggests checking the package for exact dosage guidelines.

GABA (*gamma aminobutyric acid*): One 250-milligram capsule

Calcium and magnesium: In a two-to-one ratio, such as 1,000 milligrams of calcium with 500 milligrams of magnesium

Pulsatilla: A homeopathic remedy; take as directed on the bottle

If you wake up frequently during the night, take 250 milligrams of magnesium 30 to 45 minutes before going to bed to help relax your muscles and calm your nervous system. Magnesium taken before bedtime has a tranquilizing effect on the body. Allow 1 to 2 weeks for this supplement to take effect.

Avoid eating heavy meals. Eating a lot before bedtime can make you feel bloated and gassy, thus making it more difficult to sleep peacefully.

Learn and practice regular meditations and visualization as a way to will yourself to relax.

If appropriate, take 300 milligrams of St. John's wort (*Hypericum perforatum*) three times a day. If your doctor suspects that depression is the reason for your insomnia, he may suggest St. John's wort, which is good for mild to moderate depression but not severe cases.

If all this fails, see a physician who is an expert in sleep disorders. Or visit a sleep study center, located at most of the larger medical centers.

Other Approaches

Every night, practice the basic relaxation yoga pose for 10 minutes or more before going to bed. "The basic pose will reduce the anxiety and stress that often go along with insomnia," says Judith Lasater, Ph.D., a physical therapist in San Francisco and author of *Relax and Renew*. Within an hour of your bedtime, get into the position and let your breathing prepare you for sleep, she advises.

For this pose, you need two blankets: a folded one under your neck and head and a rolled one under your knees. Lie on your back with the blankets in place, positioning your head so that your chin is slightly lower than your forehead. This position helps quiet the frontal lobes of your brain, which helps you let go of thoughts, says Dr. Lasater.

Reach out sideways, keeping your arms slightly bent and relaxed, with your palms curved upward. Relax your legs, letting your knees roll outward. Now close your eyes, swallow, let the tension drain from your lower jaw, and let your cheeks go loose. Finally, release the tension from the rest of your body, especially your shoulders, neck, and back. Maintain this relaxed position for 10 minutes or more while you inhale and exhale slowly and deeply.

Note: During pregnancy, do the basic relaxation technique while lying on your side. Use more blankets, if necessary.

Drink a cup or two of chamomile (*Matricaria recutita*) tea before going to bed. Chamomile can act like a light sedative, says Brigitte Mars, a professional member of the American Herbalists Guild and a clinical herbalist with UniTea Herbs in Boulder, Colorado. It has long been used to relax the body and mind. "You can drink one strong cup every night before bed if you would like," she says.

When thoughts of daily events keep you awake, take Coffea. Though its name suggests coffee, this homeopathic remedy can help you sleep, says Sujatha Pillai, a homeopathic physician at American WholeHealth Centers in Chicago. Another good homeopathic remedy for insomnia is Nux vomica. Follow the package directions for taking the preparations. Pillai also says that if a homeopathic remedy hasn't started to help you after 3 to 5 days, stop taking it.

Put three drops of chamomile (*Matricaria recutita*) essential oil and three drops of lavender (*Lavandula officinalis*) essential oil in a tub of warm water, and soak for an hour before bedtime. A warm bath before bed can help ease tension and stress and relax you enough to make sleep come easier, says Suzan Jaffe, Ph.D., associate adjunct professor of psychiatry and nursing at the University of Miami in Florida. By combining the warm bath with the relaxing scents of the fragrant oils, your evening ritual can be very sleep inducing.

If you have caffeinated drinks, reserve them for morning consumption. Since caffeine is a stimulant, you don't want any near bedtime, Dr. Jaffe says. If you are fond of coffee, tea, or cola, don't drink any in the afternoon and limit your daily consumption to two servings, she advises.

Avoid using alcoholic beverages to help you relax. Though people think of alcohol as a relaxant, it actually dehydrates you, which throws off the rate at which your body produces energy, says Dr. Jaffe. Drinking alcohol in the evening may help you get to sleep faster, she acknowledges, but you are more likely to wake up during the night. When morning comes, you probably won't feel rejuvenated.

Get on a regular exercise program. If you walk, bike, or swim for 30 minutes or more daily, you may have an easier time getting to sleep, says Dr. Jaffe. For best results, you should exercise in the morning or afternoon, not within 4 hours of bedtime.

Irritable Bowel Syndrome

Irritable bowel syndrome is a disorder in which the lower digestive system is not infected or inflamed but simply doesn't work in a normal manner. Sound vague? It is. In fact, doctors have not been able to find the cause of irritable bowel syndrome—yet as much as 15 percent of the population on occasion has an unexplained digestive problem that falls under the irritable bowel syndrome label. These problems can include recurring gas, bloating, abdominal pain, constipation, and diarrhea. Some believe that stress or the colon's overreaction to certain foods may be a big cause of this condition, known as IBS.

The Blended Prescription

Note: To learn about cautions and possible side effects of the remedies in this chapter, see page 253.

Irritable bowel syndrome is usually diagnosed after all other diseases of the colon are ruled out. Your doctor may check to make sure that there is no inflammation or other sign of disease by performing an endoscopy (using a flexible tube to view your colon). The doctor may also test a stool or blood sample.

There is a lot you can do to relieve IBS, much of it simple and all of it natural. Here is a seven-step prescription for effective relief, as recommended by our blended-medicine experts.

Figure out whether your diet is causing your discomfort. "People are often sensitive to foods that they don't even know they are sensitive to," says Myron B. Lezak, M.D., a gastroenterologist at the Perlmutter Health Center in Naples, Florida. Here's what to do: First, eliminate all wheat products from your diet for a week, he suggests. The following week, also eliminate dairy products.

HERBAL POWER

Peppermint for IBS

Peppermint (*Mentha piperita*) can relax both your mind and the muscles of your digestive system. Try peppermint essential oil capsules for easing problems associated with irritable bowel syndrome, recommends Myron B. Lezak, M.D., a gastroenterologist at the Perlmutter Health Center in Naples, Florida. Take one or two capsules before meals, he advises. But do not take peppermint if you have acid reflux.

"This herb is soothing to the lower gastrointestinal tract, but for it to reach there, you should take enteric-coated capsules of peppermint oil," says Andrew T. Weil, M.D., clinical professor of internal medicine and director of the integrative medicine program at the University of Arizona College of Medicine in Tucson and author of *Spontaneous Healing*. "Enteric coating resists attack by stomach acid, so the capsules pass into the intestines intact and release their contents there."

Move down the list and eliminate additional foods each week—eggs, yeast, beef, other grains, and soy. The goal is to determine if removing any of these foods from your diet brings relief. It could be one food that's the cause or a combination, so consider keeping a food diary to help identify the culprit.

Boost your fiber intake to 25 to 35 grams of fiber a day. The best sources for people with IBS are fruits and vegetables since many of these people are sensitive to grains, the other top source. You want to get both soluble and insoluble forms of fiber, and both are plentiful in fresh produce. Soluble fiber contains mucilage, a gummy substance that helps food slide through the digestive system. Insoluble fiber contains cellulose, the undigestible parts of plants that add bulk to the food moving through your digestive system.

As you increase the fiber in your diet, be sure to drink more water. Try to get eight 8-ounce glasses of water per day.

Correct any intestinal imbalances. IBS can often be aggravated by an imbalance of beneficial and harmful organisms in the intestines. "The balance of bacteria in the intestines is sometimes not given enough attention in conventional medicine," Dr. Lezak says. He recommends taking acidophilus capsules, such as those from Metagenics (available from health care professionals) and Kyo-Dophilus (available in health food stores). Follow the package directions. Yogurt with live active cultures also may be beneficial, he says, but since many people with IBS are sensitive to dairy products, first be sure that the yogurt doesn't give your gut more grief.

Learn a formal relaxation method and apply it whenever you are becoming tense or stressed. "People with IBS have bowel muscles that are very reactive to their mental states," Dr. Lezak says. It follows that stress reduction can help keep IBS at bay, but you have to work on it consistently. "Everyone has his own comfort zone for relaxation techniques," he notes. "I like meditation for 5 to 10 minutes twice a day, but some people have trouble quieting themselves for that long. In that case, they should participate in more active relaxation techniques, like yoga or tai chi. The point is to quiet the mind."

Get some exercise every day. It needn't be strenuous—an after-dinner stroll might be just the ticket. "Some people say that they need to walk every day in order to

---

SKILLFUL HEALERS

Hypnotherapy

Hypnosis may help ease anxiety, reduce pain, and improve bowel function. In a typical hypnosis session, you will be guided to a state of deep relaxation by the therapist, then asked to imagine your whole body relaxing step-by-step. The therapist will suggest thoughts of your intestines becoming immune to discomfort and disturbances. Finally, you will be brought back to a waking state.

Most researchers studying hypnosis in irritable bowel syndrome (IBS) therapy have used 30- to 40-minute sessions once every other week for 3 months, says Olafur S. Palsson, Psy.D., assistant professor of psychiatry and family medicine and director of the Behavioral Medicine Clinic at the Eastern Virginia Medical School of the Medical College of Hampton Roads in Norfolk.

"This treatment has practically no negative side effects, and it is highly effective in reducing all the central symptoms of people with IBS in at least 80 percent of severe and chronic cases," Dr. Palsson says.

have a bowel movement," says Eileen Marie Wright, M.D., a staff physician at the Great Smokies Medical Center in Asheville, North Carolina. "The bowels require some movement, but not heavy exertion. A daily 15- to 20-minute walk can make the difference."

Drink ginger (*Zingiber officinale*) tea throughout the day. Ginger's ability to ease nausea and other digestive problems is well-known. The herb can be a powerful friend to people with IBS, because it also relieves gas and spasms. Finely chop a 1-inch section of fresh ginger, add it to 2 cups of boiling water, let steep for 5 minutes, and strain. Fill an insulated container with the tea and take small sips of it throughout the day. "This tea is very soothing," Dr. Lezak says. He also likes a tea made from equal parts fennel seeds (*Foeniculum vulgare*), dried chamomile (*Matricaria recutita*), and dried peppermint (*Mentha piperita*). Prepare this the same way as you would the ginger tea.

Other Approaches

Try a Triphala supplement. Triphala is a natural supplement made from three Indian fruits, and it provides good relief for people with IBS, Dr. Wright says. It works partly as a soluble fiber and partly as a gentle stimulant, and it may help to detoxify the bowel. "If you need to take it every day, however, you are probably missing an underlying cause for your symptoms, and Triphala is not going to solve the problem," she adds. Triphala is available in health food stores. Follow the package directions.

Eat foods in their most unprocessed state. That doesn't mean you have to eat everything raw. "But it does mean that the strawberries at the bottom of a yogurt container aren't really something I would consider fruit," Dr. Wright says. "That's jam. Eat your strawberries plain." If your IBS symptoms are severe, you may want to avoid eating in restaurants. By preparing your own food, you know exactly what you are eating and are better able to avoid ingredients that trigger problems.

Jet Lag

Regulated by small cells within your brain, your internal clock helps determine when you should wake, eat, and sleep. When you switch time zones too quickly, that clock tries to stick to its normal, routine pace even while it is getting bombarded with contradictory patterns of night and day in the new time zone. The result? A fatigued, out-of-sync feeling dubbed jet lag that is very familiar to jet travelers who frequently crisscross time zones. Battered by this psychic time distortion, some people get jet lag symptoms that include headaches, irritability, insomnia, and intestinal troubles like diarrhea or constipation.

The Blended Prescription

Note: To learn about cautions and possible side effects of the remedies in this chapter, see page 253.

When you synchronize your internal clock with the new time zone, most of your jet lag problems should go away. If symptoms hang on abnormally long, see a doctor—especially if you experience leg swelling with pain on one side, shortness of breath, fatigue that won't go away, or unbearable headaches. Otherwise, here are six recommendations from our panel of blended-medicine experts to help you adjust to your new zone.

For the first five nights in the new time zone, take 1 to 3 milligrams of the hormone supplement melatonin about 30 minutes before you go to bed. Melatonin plays a key role in regulating a person's sleep cycle.

If you have traveled east, expose yourself to morning light in the new time zone. If you have traveled west, get out in the late-afternoon light. Exposure to the sun at these times will help your body readjust to the new time zone.

Use the homeopathic remedy Cocculus 6C, taking two pellets every 15 minutes for four doses, then two pellets every hour for four doses on the first day. After that, take two pellets four times a day until your symptoms are gone.

Take two pellets of Coffea 6C, another homeopathic medicine, at bedtime until symptoms resolve.

To help avoid jet lag in the first place, have 1 to 2 grams of powdered ginger (_Zingiber officinale_) in capsule form 1 hour before your flight time. Then take one capsule every hour while you are flying.

During the flight, don't drink alcoholic or caffeinated beverages (which are diuretics), and be sure to have plenty of water. The air inside an airplane's cabin is notoriously dry, and a lengthy trip can dehydrate you. Dehydration worsens jet lag, and alcohol and caffeine consumption worsens dehydration.

Other Approaches

When you get to your destination, take 150 to 300 milligrams of valerian root extract (_Valeriana officinalis_) about 30 minutes before lights-out. This herb helps you sleep by quieting the central nervous system, says Brigitte Mars, a professional member of the American Herbalists Guild and a clinical herbalist with UniTea Herbs in Boulder, Colorado. Since concentrations differ depending on the product, just follow the directions on the label.

HERBAL POWER

On Time with Ginseng

To acclimate to your new time zone more quickly, take Asian ginseng (*Panax ginseng*) or Siberian ginseng (*Eleutherococcus senticosus*) a few days before leaving for your trip and continue to take it for a few days after you arrive, says Brigitte Mars, a professional member of the American Herbalists Guild and a clinical herbalist with UniTea Herbs in Boulder, Colorado. An herb that helps the body adapt to change, ginseng helps regulate your breathing and heartbeat.

Since many different strengths are available, follow the package directions on the product you buy to take the equivalent of one dosage a day, she says.

For an aromatic sleep-inducer, mist your face with lavender-scented water. Fill a small spray bottle with 4 ounces of water, add five drops of essential oil of lavender (*Lavandula angustifolia*), and gently spray your face (be sure to close your eyes) a few times during your flight, Mars advises. After you arrive, use the mister as often as you like, and spray some lavender scent on your pillow before you go to bed. If you are concerned about the oil staining your pillowcase, cover it with an old towel.

Drink a cup of green tea when you want to stay awake. Drinking this herbal tea can invigorate you, helping you stay awake during the daylight hours in the new time zone. Just make sure that this stimulant doesn't deprive you of sleep. "I wouldn't recommend drinking more than three cups of green tea a day," says Mars.

To prevent jet lag, get plenty of rest the night before traveling. When you have a long trip coming up, try to get your packing done a day or two early so that you don't stay up late before your flight. "Most people get less sleep the night before a trip," says Suzan Jaffe, Ph.D., associate adjunct professor of psychiatry and nursing at the University of Miami in Florida. "Even when you are not changing time zones, lack of sleep can cause a pseudo jet lag."

Lactose Intolerance

Some people just can't digest lactose, or milk sugar, because they lack a milk-sugar–gobbling enzyme called lactase that the small intestine is supposed to produce. If you have an intestine that produces only a small amount of this enzyme or none at all, the undigested milk sugar gets ferried to your large intestine.

Once the milk sugar is in the large intestine, bacteria do the breakdown work, spewing out hydrogen, carbon dioxide, and organic acids in the process. As a result, someone with lactose intolerance experiences diarrhea, flatulence, bloating, and abdominal cramps within a few hours of eating dairy foods.

The Blended Prescription

Note: To learn about cautions and possible side effects of the remedies in this chapter, see page 253.

Fortunately, we now have many products that can help make up for a lack of lactase—and if you also avoid foods that cause the symptoms, you are well on your way to trouble-free dining. Here is a six-part prescription from our blended-medicine experts to help your intestinal tract with its business.

Take a daily dose of the dietary supplement Lactaid to provide the lactase that you need to digest milk sugar properly. Follow the label instructions.

Whenever you want dairy products, choose the fermented kind. You should be all right with yogurt containing live cultures, buttermilk, and hard cheeses such as Cheddar, Parmesan, Swiss, and Jarlsberg. The bacteria used in fermentation produce a lactase to digest the lactose.

Substitute soy milk, rice milk, or oat milk for regular milk. Also, eat frozen products like Rice Dream instead of ice cream or frozen yogurt. Instead of regular soft cheese, have soy cheese.

If you try any dairy foods that might contain lactose, always have them with meals in order to reduce symptoms.

Eat high-calcium foods. Try spinach, broccoli, calcium-fortified orange juice, and tofu. In addition, take 800 milligrams a day of a calcium supplement. This is to replace the calcium you would have gotten in dairy foods.

Twice a day, stir 1 teaspoon of nondairy acidophilus powder in a glass of water and drink. It will encourage the growth of "good" bacteria in your digestive system.

Laryngitis

The larynx is a delicate apparatus that can easily be thrown out of kilter. Catch a nasty cold or flu, scream too loud at your kids (or your spouse), or hit the highest octave of your favorite ballad one time too many, and you can end up with laryngitis, inflammation of the vocal cords. Once they are inflamed, your throat may feel raw and may tickle, and your voice may take on the rasp of Don Corleone from *The Godfather* or the high-pitched squeal of Tweety bird from Looney Tunes. Or you may lose your voice completely.

The Blended Prescription

Note: To learn about cautions and possible side effects of the remedies in this chapter, see page 253.

You should see a doctor if your laryngitis has silenced you for more than a week or if it came on very suddenly (within a few minutes to half an hour), which could mean

---

SKILLFUL HEALERS

Reflexology

A reflexologist might stimulate the throat/neck reflex points on your feet to relieve throat congestion and the spleen points on your feet to stimulate your immune system, says Laura Norman, a licensed massage therapist, a leading reflexology authority in New York City, and author of *Feet First: A Guide to Foot Reflexology*. Another possible area for stimulation is the pituitary gland region, to get your endocrine glands up to speed.

If the reflexologist works on the diaphragm and adrenal gland areas in the middle of your foot, the session can help reduce throat inflammation, says Norman. Pressing the tops and base of your toes clears sinus and nasal passages and helps release blocked energy and bloodflow from your shoulders and neck to your head, she adds.

Reflexology proponents believe these sessions improve circulation to the throat area, help fight infection, and help eliminate toxins in the body.

that your vocal cords are bruised. Most doctors prescribe antibiotics if your laryngitis is caused by a bacterial infection. Otherwise, treating this condition is up to you.

Here are four all-natural approaches to laryngitis relief, as prescribed by our team of blended-medicine experts.

Take 50,000 international units (IU) of beta-carotene and 2,000 milligrams of vitamin C three times a day until your symptoms subside. These large doses give your immune system the jump start it needs to remedy your vocal cords.

Three times a day, between meals, take two 375-milligram capsules of bromelain at a potency of 2,400 mcu (a standard unit of measurement for enzymes) until symptoms subside. Bromelain is an enzyme found in pineapple that helps treat inflammation and increases circulation.

Using supplement capsules, take 200 milligrams of echinacea (*Echinacea purpurea*) or goldenseal (*Hydrastis canadensis*) or both, four times a day for at least 2 weeks. These two herbal extracts help to bolster the body's immune system.

For homeopathic relief, take two pellets of Argentum nitricum 6C, Aconitum napellus 6C, or Spongia tosta 6C. Take the pellets every 15 minutes for four doses, followed by two pellets every hour for four doses on the first day. After that, take two pellets every 6 hours until your symptoms subside.

Other Approaches

Inhale the vapors of eucalyptus (*Eucalyptus globulus*) and peppermint (*Mentha piperita*) two or three times a day, depending on the severity of your symptoms. Bring 3 cups of water to a boil, remove from the stove, and add fresh or dried eucalyptus and peppermint leaves. Make an inhalation tent by draping a towel over your head, and breathe in the steam from a comfortable distance.

Place two drops each of cypress (*Cupressus semper-virens*), sandalwood (*Santalum album*), lavender (*Lavandula vera*), and cedarwood (*Cedrus atlantica*) essential oils in a sterile bottle with ½ ounce of olive or sweet almond oil. Shake the mixture, then massage a few drops as needed into the front of your neck so that it penetrates the skin, enters the bloodstream, and starts working to alleviate symptoms, suggests Ixchel Leigh, an aromatherapist and regional director of the National Association for Holistic Aromatherapy in Durango, Colorado.

All these essential oils possess antibacterial, antiseptic, antispasmodic, and anti-inflammatory properties that fight infection, break up congestion, suppress coughing, and reduce pain and inflammation, says Leigh.

Use a wet wrap around your neck. Wet a washcloth with cold water, wring it out, and fold it over twice to form a long rectangle, suggests Michael Traub, N.D., a naturopathic physician in Kailua Kona, Hawaii. Drape the washcloth around your neck and cover it with a dry towel, wool scarf, or muffler. Leave it there for about 20 minutes, letting it heat up. As the wet washcloth gets warm, it encourages blood circulation and white blood cell migration to your neck, helping to fight infection, he explains. You can remove the wrap after 20 minutes, wet it again, and repeat the procedure as often as you like, he says.

Menopause

If you are a woman, your levels of the hormones estrogen and progesterone begin to decline as you move through your forties and fifties. The hormone deprivation causes a domino effect that alters menstruation patterns as well as mood and body temperature, and it causes a host of other physical and emotional changes. At times, you might become so hot that your hair and clothes get wet with sweat. And you may experience fatigue, vaginal dryness, moodiness, and irregular bleeding, to name just a few symptoms. Few of these changes pass quickly; they sometimes go on for years both before and after your last period.

The Blended Prescription

Note: To learn about cautions and possible side effects of the remedies in this chapter, see page 253.

To cope with some problems associated with "the change," first consider your diet. From there, possible treatments run the gamut from herbs to homeopathic remedies to hormone-replacement therapy. Here are five steps for relief, as suggested by our panel of blended-medicine experts.

Take 400 international units (IU) of vitamin E in capsules twice a day. Vitamin E helps to stabilize erratic blood vessel walls that cause hot flashes. You should notice the effects of vitamin E within a few weeks or months. Continue taking it even after menopause has subsided. If you decide to stop taking vitamin E after a period of time, monitor the frequency of your hot flashes. This may help you decide whether or not to resume vitamin E therapy.

Two times each day, take a 40-milligram supplement of black cohosh (*Actea racemosa*). Continue taking the herb even after menopause is over. Black cohosh acts like the hormone estrogen in the body and has a long history of usage for menstrual and menopausal discomfort. If you decide to stop taking black cohosh, monitor the frequency of your symptoms. This may help you to decide whether or not to resume black cohosh therapy.

Supplement with 100 milligrams of Siberian ginseng (*Eleutherococcus senticosus*) twice daily. Ginseng can help relieve fatigue and hot flashes and can possibly have a positive effect on slight depression. Keep taking Siberian ginseng even after menopause has subsided.

Twice a day, have 225 milligrams of chasteberry (*Vitex agnus-castus*). Chasteberry is believed to help stabilize the female sex hormones. If you decide to stop taking chasteberry after a period of time, monitor the frequency of your menopausal symptoms. This may help you decide whether or not to resume chasteberry therapy.

If you experience heavy menstrual bleeding, hot flashes, and feelings of irritability, try the homeopathic medicine Lachesis 6C. Take two pellets every 15 minutes until the symptoms subside, then reduce the dose to two pellets every 4 hours for four doses on the first day. After that, change the potency to 30C and take two pellets each day as needed until symptoms subside.

Other Approaches

Take Sepia 6X or 30C to relieve night sweats and heavy periods. Sepia can be taken once every 3 to 4 hours if symptoms are mild or as often as every 5 minutes if symptoms are severe, says Paula G. Maas, D.O., M.D., a homeopathic doctor, chairman of primary care at the Touro University College of Osteopathic Medicine in San Francisco, and coauthor of *Natural Medicine for Menopause and Beyond*. Choose the frequency of doses depending on your symptoms. Continue to use Sepia until your symptoms resolve.

When you feel fatigued, lie on the floor and rock forward and backward on your spine. With the pressure on your back, you are essentially using acupressure to help balance your energy to fight the fatigue that can go along with menopause, says Dr. Maas.

If you don't have a carpeted floor, cushion your back with an exercise mat or blanket. Lie on your back and bring your knees close to your chest. Rock back until your shoulders touch the floor, then immediately rock forward again. Continue rocking back and forth until your feelings of fatigue pass, Dr. Maas says.

If you are looking for a magic pill that could make your menopause symptoms go away, hormone-replacement therapy (HRT) might be what you want. When you get hormone therapy, you are replacing the declining estrogen supplies in your body, says Gregory Burke, M.D., professor and vice chairman of the department of public health sciences at the Bowman Gray School of Medicine of Wake Forest University in Winston-Salem, North Carolina.

Because every woman is different, it is very important that HRT be tailored to your symptoms and hormone levels. If you think HRT is for you, see your family doctor, gynecologist, or internist about therapy options.

Motion Sickness

Travel by car, plane, boat, or train. It doesn't matter. The bouncing, bobbing, dipping, and swaying motion can cause your eyes, sensory nerves, and inner ear to send mismatched messages to your brain about the movement affecting your body. As a result, your brain becomes confused, your stomach feels queasy, and your head starts spinning. Fatigue, sweating, faintness, and breathing difficulties often follow.

The Blended Prescription

Note: To learn about cautions and possible side effects of the remedies in this chapter, see page 253.

The best cure for motion sickness is to prevent it or nip early symptoms in the bud—fast. This simple four-step plan from our blended-medicine experts is for prevention and relief.

Take two 500-milligram capsules of powdered ginger (*Zingiber officinale*) about 30 minutes before you travel. Then swallow one or two more capsules about every 4 hours as needed. Ginger is touted as one of the best antinausea remedies around. Researchers speculate it works by blocking the body's nausea signals and vomiting reflexes, says William D. Nelson, N.D., a naturopathic physician in Colorado Springs, Colorado.

You can also eat candied ginger (available at Asian markets and health food stores) and drink fresh ginger tea 2 hours before travel and every 3 to 4 hours en route.

Take an over-the-counter remedy that contains dimenhydrinate (Dramamine) or meclizine (Bonine). For dosing instructions, follow the package directions. Transderm

---

HERBAL POWER

Calm with Peppermint

Fragrant peppermint can do more than just delight your tastebuds; it can settle your stomach, too.

Peppermint (*Mentha piperita*) has antispasmodic properties that can calm queasiness, says Chris Meletis, N.D., professor of natural pharmacology and nutrition, dean of clinical education, and chief medical officer at the National College of Naturopathic Medicine in Portland, Oregon.

Drink a cup of peppermint tea 1 to 1½ hours before traveling and another cup 1 hour into your journey if needed. You can also take two 500-milligram peppermint capsules 1 hour before your trip and one capsule every 2 hours during the trip.

Scop is a prescription alternative. It comes as a patch that slowly releases the drug scopolamine through your skin over a 3-day period.

These medications work by shutting down nausea messages traveling to the brain via the central nervous system. They work best when taken or applied before you travel.

Essential oils can be particularly effective in treating certain symptoms of motion sickness. Lavender (*Lavandula angustifolia*), Roman chamomile (*Chamaemelum nobile*), lemon (*Citrus limon*), lemongrass (*Cymbopogon citratus*), peppermint (*Mentha piperita*), and ginger (*Zingiber officinale*) may be used for stomach upsets from motion sickness, according to Haley Zee, an aromatherapist and president of Haley Zee Associates, an aromatherapy consulting firm and product manufacturer in Leucadia, California. Lavender, lemon, and ginger are very effective for nausea. Lavender, Roman chamomile, and lemongrass are best for headaches. People with nervous tension should try lavender, Roman chamomile, lemongrass, or peppermint.

Mix three or four drops of the essential oil into 1 ounce of vegetable or canola oil. As you begin your journey, apply a few drops of this mixture under your nostrils and around your sinus area. This procedure may be performed repeatedly. Or place one of these essential oils (three or four drops per 1 ounce of water) in an atomizer to spray on your hands. "When these oils are inhaled or applied as a mist, they give you an instant feeling of well-being and relief," says Zee.

Drink plenty of fluids (other than alcohol or caffeinated beverages) during travel. This will keep your digestive system flushed and healthy. Dehydration can worsen motion sickness.

Other Approaches

Place your index fingers just below your earlobes in the indentations behind your jawbone. To balance your inner-ear message centers, apply *light* pressure while breathing deeply for 1 to 2 minutes. Repeat two more times if necessary, says David Field, N.D., a naturopathic physician and licensed acupuncturist in Santa Rosa, California.

To help calm your nerves and reduce nausea, try acupressure wristbands. Available at drugstores and travel goods stores, the wristbands can be placed on a strategic point three finger-widths from the center of your wrist to stimulate a meridian pathway that can prevent and alleviate nausea. The bands stabilize the imbalances that a motion-sensitive person experiences, says Chris Meletis, N.D., professor of natural pharmacology and nutrition, dean of clinical education, and chief medical officer at the National College of Naturopathic Medicine in Portland, Oregon.

Eat low-fat, high-carbohydrate foods such as breads, crackers, and cereals before traveling. These foods soak up stomach acid, which plays a major role in causing motion sickness, says Dr. Nelson. Avoid heavy, high-fat fare and gas-producing foods such as beans. They have a tendency to just sit in your stomach, distend your intestinal tract, and add to the misery.

Muscle Cramps

Muscles normally contract to do a task and relax when the movement is completed. With a cramp, the muscle contracts into a tight knot and doesn't relax again on its own.

Why? Nerves send muscles signals for when to contract and relax. If there is too little calcium, magnesium, hormones, body fluids, or oxygen in the blood, the signals' transmission can get tangled. The muscle responds by cramping. A variety of factors can deplete these important substances: overexertion, inadequate intake of fluids when it's hot, smoking, inactivity, and oral contraceptives, to name a few.

The Blended Prescription

Note: To learn about cautions and possible side effects of the remedies in this chapter, see page 253.

If muscle cramps occur frequently, if pain is severe, or if there is swelling, see your doctor. That said, most cramps are singular events. For periodic cramps, this six-part prescription from our blended-medicine experts tells how to get instant relief and then prevent recurrences.

Stretch and gently massage the muscle immediately. This is the fastest technique for relieving cramped muscles, says Steven Subotnick, D.P.M., N.D., Ph.D., clinical professor of biomechanics and surgery at the California College of Podiatric Medicine in Hayward, a specialist in sports medicine, and author of *Sports and Exercise Injuries*. If you awaken with a calf muscle cramp at night, for instance, simply getting out of bed onto your feet will stretch the muscle enough to ease the pain. You might also want to pace around your bedroom a little.

Apply heat to the muscle to draw blood and nutrients to it. Either use a moist, warmed towel or step into a comfortably hot bath or shower.

Apply arnica (*Arnica montana*) ointment as often as needed, following the package instructions. This popular

HERBAL POWER

Black Cohosh

Black cohosh (*Actea racemosa*) is a natural sedative that can help ease persistent muscle cramps. It comes as tincture, syrup, capsules, fluid extract, and powder. As a tincture, take 30 to 40 drops every 3 to 6 hours until cramping subsides, says John Collins, N.D., a naturopathic physician and a teacher of homeopathy at the National College of Naturopathic Medicine in Portland, Oregon. For whatever form you buy, follow the dosage directions on the package.

herbal medicine is commonly used to reduce swelling and relieve the pain of bumps, bruises, and cramps.

Take two pellets of Cuprum metallicum 6C every 15 minutes until the spasm subsides, then two pellets every 4 hours until the spasm is completely gone. This homeopathic remedy can stop a muscle contraction almost immediately, says Dr. Subotnick. Whenever the pain moves in, pop a dose under your tongue and let it dissolve.

To keep your muscles free of spasms, take the following supplements.

Calcium: 1,000 milligrams per day. Calcium is important for proper muscle contraction and release as well as for its better-known attribute of promoting strong teeth and bones.

Magnesium: Up to 500 milligrams per day. This is another mineral that is beneficial for proper muscle function, says David Edelberg, M.D., assistant professor of medicine at Rush Medical College in Chicago and founder of the American WholeHealth Centers in Chicago, Boston, Denver, and Bethesda, Maryland.

Vitamin E: Up to 800 international units (IU) per day. Vitamin E helps improve general circulation and keeps your muscles supplied with what they need to work well, says Dr. Subotnick.

If calf cramps repeatedly awaken you at night, see a doctor about getting a prescription for quinine. An alkaloid, quinine has muscle-relaxing and painkilling properties.

Other Approaches

Consider another homeopathic remedy: Magnesium phosphorica 6X. Also known as Mag phos, this remedy is made from magnesium and phosphate, both important in muscle and nervous function, says Dr. Subotnick. Homeopathic doctors recommend this remedy if your cramps feel better with heat and hard pressure. Available in health food stores, this remedy works well when dissolved in warm water and taken before bed. So heat up a glass of bottled water (tap water is not recommended because of possible metal contamination), dissolve the dose in it, stir, and sip until it's gone. Take four pellets twice a day until you feel relief, Dr. Subotnick recommends. ·

Take a warm bath before bed, particularly if you are susceptible to nighttime muscle cramps. The warm bath improves your circulation and supplies your muscles and nerves with much-needed nutrients and oxygen, says Dale Anderson, M.D., clinical assistant professor at the University of Minnesota Medical School in Minneapolis and author of *Muscle Pain Relief in 90 Seconds: The Fold and Hold Method.* An hour or so before bed, fill the tub with warm water and soak for 15 to 20 minutes.

Neck Pain

When a 10-pound sphere is supported by a skinny stalk of muscle and bone, it is a setup for trouble. And trouble arrives in the form of neck pain when your pillow's not right, when you hit the brakes too hard at a stoplight, or when you tense up because of stress. Your neck muscles go into spasm. And when you hunch your shoulders to help support your head, the pain gets worse— even leading to headaches in some cases.

The Blended Prescription

Note: To learn about cautions and possible side effects of the remedies in this chapter, see page 253.

In most cases, neck pain should not be cause for alarm unless the pain is accompanied by severe headache, nausea, vomiting, light sensitivity, drowsiness, confusion, or fever. These symptoms may signal the possibility of meningitis or brain hemorrhage, and you should seek emergency care immediately. For ordinary neck pain, your best bet is to prevent the causes, particularly if your sleeping habits are causing the kink. But when pain hits, there is much you can do to relax the muscles. Here is a seven-step prescription from our blended-medicine experts to do just that.

When neck muscles feel strained, place your chin on your chest to stretch the muscles to their full length. Then reach behind your head and gently but firmly massage all the muscles in your neck. Move your fingers in small circles about the size of a dime, traveling from your shoulders up the base of your skull. Since the neck muscles extend over your skull, include your scalp and forehead in this massage.

If you have the time, make a relaxing massage oil. Use a neutral carrier oil, such as almond, to which you add a few drops of essential oil of lavender (*Lavandula*, various species).

Take the homeopathic painkiller Arnica 6C. Take two pellets every 15 minutes until the pain lessens, then two pellets every 4 hours until the pain is completely gone. In addition, you can rub arnica (*Arnica montana*) ointment into the painful area, following the directions on the label. This pain-relieving ointment is derived from arnica flowers and is an age-old herbal remedy available at most health food stores.

Take an 800-milligram supplement of the muscle-friendly mineral magnesium each day when neck pain is an issue. Magnesium has the ability to draw water from inflamed muscles and tissue, easing the pain.

Take a nonsteroidal anti-inflammatory pain reliever like ibuprofen. If massage and relaxation don't kill the pain or inflammation, this probably will. Use as directed on the bottle.

If neck pain is associated with stress or anxiety, consider taking a calming herb. Try kava kava (*Piper methysticum*), skullcap (*Scutellaria lateriflora*), hops (*Humulus lupulus*), or passionflower (*Passiflora incarnata*). Steep 2 teaspoons of one of these dry herbs in hot water for 10 minutes to bring out its medicinal qualities. Strain, then drink three or four times a day as needed. Or get capsules of the standardized extract and follow the package instructions.

For neck pain that radiates from the base of your skull, try a homemade acupressure device. Called a de-tenniser because it is made with two tennis balls, this device was dreamed up by Dale Anderson, M.D., clinical assistant professor at the University of Minnesota Medical School in Minneapolis and author of *Muscle Pain Relief in 90 Seconds:*

The Fold and Hold Method. Besides two tennis balls, you will also need an old pair of panty hose. Here's how to make it.

1. Cut off one leg near the top. Cut off the foot portion of the leg. You'll have an opening on both ends.
2. Slip the two balls into the stocking leg and slide them together in the middle of the leg.
3. Tie two knots in the stocking, snugly against each tennis ball, leaving 1- to 2-foot stocking tails on each side.

To use your de-tenniser, lie on your back on a firm surface such as a carpeted floor, exercise mat, or throw rug. Place the de-tenniser behind your neck so the two balls are positioned where the soft muscles meet the hard skull. Let your neck relax so the entire weight is resting in between the balls. If you like, you can increase the pressure a bit by gripping the loose ends of the stocking and pulling upward gently.

Relax in this position for 90 seconds, letting the top of your head drop toward the floor as far as possible while allowing your chin to move toward the ceiling. Very slowly, come out of the position and sit up.

You can repeat this acupressure technique whenever necessary to relieve neck discomfort.

Note: Consult your doctor before performing this exercise if you are over age 65 or have vascular problems, circulatory problems, or arthritis in your neck. Also consult your doctor if arching your neck backward causes lightheadedness or dizziness.

Other Approaches

Try out a new pillow. If you wake up with neck pain, your pillow might be crunching your neck while it is cradling your head. Often, changing your pillow is a way to relieve pain, says Joseph Smith, D.C., a chiropractor

SKILLFUL HEALERS

Chiropractic

The technique many people refer to as having your neck cracked is actually called manipulation. Performed by a qualified expert, chiropractic manipulation may be just the ticket to setting you free from your stiff neck.

Chiropractic manipulation is a completely passive healing modality, says Joseph Smith, D.C., a chiropractor with Chiropractic Associates in Fogelsville, Pennsylvania. "The most important thing for the patient to do is relax," he says. That's because manipulation works through the adjustment of vertebrae in the back and neck. These tiny, specific adjustments are made by the skilled hands of your chiropractor.

The movements are quick and to the point. And the procedure is usually painless. "It can feel very comfortable, even relaxing," says Dr. Smith. "But, of course, it varies on the condition you have to start with." While you may require more than one treatment for complete healing, immediate relief of pain and restoration of some range of motion is a definite possibility.

with Chiropractic Associates in Fogelsville, Pennsylvania. If you are sleeping on two pillows, maybe you need just one—or you might need a flatter pillow rather than a fluffy one. Try out pillows that are made from different contents, which affects their firmness. Water, foam, and feather pillows are all available, and you can even find some that have a filling made from buckwheat hulls. "This is probably one of the simplest ways to address neck pain," Dr. Smith says. "And it's definitely worth a try." Be sure to test the new pillow for two or three nights—long enough to give it a real try.

Keep away from cold air and drafts when sleeping. Although chilly drafts won't give you a runny nose, they can lock up your neck. "Cold air—whether it's from an open window or an air conditioner—makes your neck muscles contract," says Dr. Smith. "If you happen to be sleeping in an unusual position, the muscles tighten around your neck joints and compress them."

If you like to keep a window open at night, move your bed so that the breeze doesn't blow directly over your pillow. If you are using an air conditioner and are waking with a stiff neck, try turning the unit's dial to the lowest possible setting. Or move your bed farther away from the source of the cool-air draft.

Nosebleeds

The skin inside your nose is lined with a network of thin, fragile capillaries that deliver blood and oxygen. These tiny vessels are no match for the forced-air pressure that you create when you blow your nose. If you sustain the blowout too long or too hard, these capillaries can burst, releasing their caches of blood. Or maybe dry air is the problem. When your nasal vessels harden and dry, just the touch of a tissue could make them crack open and leak out drops of blood. An unexpected jab and blood-thinning medicines can also cause nosebleeds.

The Blended Prescription

Note: To learn about cautions and possible side effects of the remedies in this chapter, see page 253.

Severe bleeding or bleeding that lasts more than 20 minutes should send a signal to your common sense: Call

HERBAL POWER

A "Berry" Good Herb

Bilberry extract (*Vaccinium myrtillus*) is a natural medicine known for decreasing the fragility of small blood vessels and preventing nosebleeds, says Jennifer Brett, N.D., a naturopathic physician in Norwalk and Stratford, Connecticut. Take two 60-milligram capsules a day to prevent nosebleeds.

Blueberries and raspberries are just as effective as bilberry extract, she adds. So including about 1 cup of either fresh blueberries or raspberries in your diet every day will help fend off nosebleeds.

your doctor or visit the emergency room to find out what is causing it. But you can halt most nosebleeds safely and swiftly by adhering to this simple four-step prescription from our blended-medicine experts.

With your head tilted forward—not backward—firmly pinch the area of your nose just below where the hard nasal bone changes into soft cartilage. Apply either an ice pack wrapped in a thin towel or a washcloth soaked in ice water and wrung out to the back of your neck. Why not lean backward, as so many mothers would tell you? Leaning forward gets gravity to work in getting blood and mucus out of your nose. And if you lean forward, you won't get blood down the back of your throat, says Alan J. Sogg, M.D., an otolaryngologist in Cleveland.

If the bleeding continues for more than 5 minutes, use a nasal decongestant spray or saline nasal spray. These sprays tighten up the capillaries and seal the bloodflow, says Jennifer Brett, N.D., a naturopathic physician in Norwalk and Stratford, Connecticut. Spray once in each nostril. To make a quick anti-nosebleed solution, stir 1 teaspoon of salt into a cup of water warmed to body temperature until the salt dissolves. Pour some of this solution into your hand, then inhale two or three times per nostril to "snuffle" it into your nose.

Another method: Squirt the decongestant or concentrated salt solution on a cotton ball, wring out the excess liquid, and then gently insert the cotton into the bleeding nostril, says Dr. Sogg. Pinch your nostrils together and breathe through your mouth for 5 minutes. Keep the cotton ball in for another 30 minutes before carefully removing it.

Make a yarrow tea. First, make a cup of the tea that you normally drink. Then add 1 tablespoon of dried yarrow (*Achillea millefolium*), steep for 5 minutes, strain, and drink. If there is leftover yarrow tea, cool it with an ice cube and soak a piece of soft cloth in it. Wring out the cloth, place it over the bridge of your nose, and pinch. Hold it in place for 5 to 10 minutes. Yarrow works much like a natural decongestant, says Dr. Brett. It constricts blood vessels and helps clotting.

Consider using a homeopathic medicine to halt the bloodflow. Choices include Ferrum phosphoricum (when a nosebleed comes after injury) or Hamamelis (when a nosebleed comes after sneezing). Take two pellets of 6C potency every 15 minutes until bleeding stops.

Other Approaches

To prevent nosebleeds, blow more softly. "Take a normal breath in and out when you blow your nose," Dr. Brett says. "If you are blowing to the point that your ears pop, you are blowing too hard."

Invest in a humidifier for your home. This machine pumps moisture into the air, which is especially dry in winter. In fact, winter is the time when you run the greatest risk of nosebleeds, notes Dr. Sogg.

Rub liquid vitamin E in your nostrils. Puncture a gel capsule with a needle, squeeze out one or two drops of vitamin E oil, and rub the oil inside your nostrils. Lubricated with the oil, your capillaries will be less likely to break during dry weather or if you have a cold, says Dr. Brett. Using one or two drops of coconut oil can produce the same effect, she adds.

Take 1,000 milligrams of vitamin C with bioflavonoids twice a day. This supplement can bolster the strength of your nasal blood vessels, says Dr. Brett.

Sniff excess mucus into your throat and spit it out. If you are outdoors or near a bathroom, spit out excess mucus instead of blowing your nose, advises Dr. Sogg. This protects your nose capillaries from frequent nose blowing.

Oily Hair

Beneath your scalp, sebaceous glands attached to hair follicles pump out an oily substance called sebum. Sebum is key to healthy hair. But a high-fat diet, a hormone imbalance, or stress can shift oil glands into overdrive, causing greasy, limp locks.

The Blended Prescription

Note: To learn about cautions and possible side effects of the remedies in this chapter, see page 253.

Oily hair can be a sign of thyroid or adrenal disease, so see your doctor if it doesn't clear up after using these remedies for 6 weeks.

Eating a low-fat diet that's high in fruits and vegetables can reduce oiliness in your hair and skin. After that, try the following four-step prescription from our blended-medicine experts.

Every morning, mix 1 tablespoon of flaxseed (*Linum usitatissimum*) oil into yogurt or juice. Flaxseed oil is a good source of essential fatty acids, which tend to normalize sebum production.

For a nourishing scalp treatment, mix five drops of rosemary (*Rosmarinus officinalis*) essential oil and five drops of elemi (*Canarium luzonicum*) essential oil into 1 ounce of jojoba (*Simmonsia chinensis*) oil. Massage 1 tablespoon of the oils into your scalp before bedtime. To protect your pillow, put a towel over it while sleeping. Wash your hair as usual in the morning. Repeat the treatment at least twice weekly. This blend can be added to any shampoo.

Put 8 ounces of aloe vera juice and two drops each of lemon (*Citrus limon*), ylang-ylang (*Cananga odorata*), and geranium (*Pelargonium roseum*) essential oils in a misting bottle. Shake well, then mist daily into your freshly washed hair and massage into your scalp. This mixture decreases oil production and promotes healthy hair.

The following blend of vitamins and supplements maximizes hair health and helps put a halt to oil production.

Vitamin A: Take 50,000 international units (IU) daily for 3 weeks, then reduce your intake to 10,000 IU each day.

B-complex vitamin: Take one tablet of B-complex 50 each morning and evening, plus 50 milligrams of vitamin B_6 each morning.

Borage (Borago officinalis) oil: Take one 1,000-milligram capsule, which gives you about 240 milligrams of gamma-linolenic acid (GLA), each morning.

PABA (*para-aminobenzoic acid*): Take 500 milligrams a day for a month.

Oily Skin

When you were a teenager, hyperactive sebaceous glands tucked beneath your skin cranked out an overabundance of an oily substance called sebum. For most people, merely growing up brought an end to that problem. But for some adults, excessive sebum creation remains a problem. The cause is often hereditary or hormonal, but it could also be dietary. The substance of sebum is actually waste by-products—some of the leftovers from your energy-burning body. When your diet is too high in saturated fats, your body can't burn up the fats very efficiently, so more leftover waste seeps to the surface, carried in the sebum.

The Blended Prescription

Note: To learn about cautions and possible side effects of the remedies in this chapter, see page 253.

Oily skin can be a sign of thyroid or adrenal disease, so see your doctor if your oily skin doesn't clear up after using these remedies for 6 weeks. You should also see a doctor if your oily skin is accompanied by unusual constipation, weight gain, or fatigue.

Proper cleaning is an obvious solution to oily skin. By proper, we mean gentle cleaning with gentle ingredients, such as witch hazel or prepackaged facial wipes from skin care companies. To get to the root of the problem, however, you need to get below the surface of the skin. Here is a six-step program of foods and supplements to help diminish your skin's oil production, as prescribed by our team of blended-medicine experts.

Eat a diet with a lot of fresh fruits and vegetables—and stay away from red meat, fried foods, full-fat dairy products, shortening, and other hydrogenated vegetable oils. The goal is to reduce your intake of saturated fats to 10 percent of your calories by replacing fatty foods with healthier, nutrient-rich foods.

Have one tablet of B-complex 50 twice a day. If it is effective, you can continue to take this as part of your daily regimen. The B-complex vitamins include thiamin, riboflavin, niacin, pantothenic acid, vitamin B_6, vitamin B_{12}, folic acid, and biotin. B vitamins help you metabolize fats better so that you use them as an energy source instead of eliminating them through sebum.

Take 50,000 international units (IU) of vitamin A every day for 3 weeks, then reduce the dose to 10,000 IU per day. Vitamin A helps to dry out the skin. In fact, too much vitamin A in a person's diet can cause dry skin.

Add 1 tablespoonful of flaxseed (*Linum usitatissimum*) oil to your yogurt or juice every morning. Flaxseed oil, a good source of essential fatty acids, helps to normalize sebum production.

Each morning, swallow one 1,000-milligram capsule of borage (*Borago officinalis*) oil. This gives you about 240 milligrams of gamma-linolenic acid (GLA), which works much the same way as B vitamins to help you metabolize fats better.

Take the homeopathic remedy Natrum muriaticum 6C in the form of two pellets four times a day for 2 to 3 weeks. If it is effective, you can continue taking it indefinitely at a dosage of two pellets each morning. Homeopaths use this remedy to treat a variety of skin ailments, including boils and painful acne.

Other Approaches

Take 250 milligrams of the B vitamin pantothenic acid every morning. That's in addition to the B-complex supplement recommended above. Pantothenic acid plays an important role in adrenal gland function. You will produce less adrenaline when you are stressed, and with less adrenaline secretion, you produce less sebum, says Jennifer Brett, N.D., a naturopathic physician in Norwalk and Stratford, Connecticut.

Gently wash your face two or three times a day. You may be tempted to scrub that oil away every chance you get. But washing your face too often—more than three times a day—may stimulate your skin to produce more oil. "Every skin pore is a little oil factory," says Mary Lupo, M.D., associate clinical professor of dermatology at Tulane University School of Medicine in New Orleans. "Your skin knows how much oil is produced, as if it had a little dipstick. So if you constantly remove that oil, your skin says, 'Oops, not enough oil. Better make some more.'" Hard scrubbing and rubbing stir up the oil glands, too, so be gentle.

Wash with antibacterial soap. Avoid superfatted soaps (like Dove and Tone), which are intended to moisturize as they clean. Your skin doesn't need any added oil. "Antibacterial soaps (like Dial and Lever 2000) are helpful," says Susan C. Taylor, M.D., assistant clinical professor of medicine in the department of dermatology at the University of Pennsylvania School of Medicine in Philadelphia. That's because oily skin has a tendency to clog the pores and foster bacterial growth.

Overweight

More than half of U.S. adults are overweight. The how of weight gain is simple: If you take in more calories than you burn, the excess gets converted into fat. The why of weight gain is more complicated. Numerous factors come into play, many of them highly individualized: how efficiently your body burns calories, when you eat, what your genetic makeup is, what role food plays in your mental well-being. Experts also point to a sedentary lifestyle as another reason American bellies are bursting.

The Blended Prescription

Note: To learn about cautions and possible side effects of the remedies in this chapter, see page 253.

"My theme in the post–Fen-phen era is 'Back to the Future,'" says G. Michael Steelman, M.D., chairman of the board of trustees of the American Society of Bariatric Physicians, referring to headline news in 1997 that a popular combination of weight-loss drugs termed Fen-phen had serious side effects. "Eat right, get moderate exercise—that always has been and always will be the mainstay of weight loss." Sounds simple, no? But there is more that you can do, ranging from metabolism-bolstering spices to minerals that help your body store less fat. Here is a seven-step prescription for weight loss from our blended-medicine experts that mixes the tried and true with some ideas that you might not have seen before.

Sharply increase your daily water intake. Water helps you feel full, and it helps remove the wastes that fatty tissue generates when you exercise. Whatever you are drinking, double it, recommends Jennifer Brett, N.D., a naturopathic physician in Norwalk and Stratford, Connecticut. Those with heart or kidney problems, however, should consult their doctors first, since the extra water could put undue pressure on these organs. Don't sabotage your efforts by eating sugar or drinking caffeinated beverages such as tea, coffee, and colas. Both sugar and caffeine act as diuretics and cause you to urinate more.

Eat something every few hours throughout the day. Your body reacts to long periods of no food by slowing down its metabolism and conserving energy; the result is slower weight loss. By eating regularly, your body burns calories more aggressively.

Of course, that doesn't mean eat *more*. It means spreading out your food intake so you avoid that traditional big dinner. In fact, make breakfast your largest meal of the day and dinner your smallest. This gives you more energy during the

---

HERBAL POWER

A Ginseng Craving

Ginseng—be it American, Siberian, or Asian (*Panax quinquefolius, Eleutherococcus senticosus,* or *P. ginseng,* respectively)—can help you fight the cravings and reduce the stress that can sabotage weight loss. The craving for sweets is universal, and herbs that help balance blood sugar tend to help fight those cravings, explains Jennifer Brett, N.D., a naturopathic physician in Norwalk and Stratford, Connecticut. The best-known herb for this, she says, is ginseng.

Ginseng also helps to reduce stress. "In my office, the number one reason people overindulge in food is as a stress-reduction technique. If you can curb the feelings of stress, chances are you won't overeat," says Dr. Brett. She recommends taking three or four capsules, each containing 400 to 600 milligrams of ginseng root, daily. Take them between meals to help fight your cravings for sweets.

day so you won't be as tempted to eat sugary snacks and drink caffeinated beverages to keep yourself alert.

Limit both sugar and saturated fat in your diet. While excess saturated fat has been the target of choice for dieters for 2 decades, sugar is also an important culprit. Refined sugar is extremely high in empty calories and plays havoc with your metabolism. So when looking at food labels, look at sugar grams as well as saturated fat grams, and try to minimize both.

Eat "whole" foods—that is, foods in their entire, unprocessed form. Examples are fruits, vegetables, beans, and brown rice. They have little fat. They have lots of fiber, which fills you up quickly and aids your digestion. They contain loads of minerals and vitamins essential to a healthy weight and overall health. And they keep you away from processed foods that have the exact opposite attributes.

Consider taking water-soluble fiber supplements, such as psyllium. Water-soluble fiber supplements, when combined with water, make your stomach feel full. In addition, they reduce the number of calories the body can absorb, by keeping food moving quickly through the digestive tract. Psyllium is found in commercial bulk laxatives, such as Metamucil. Take 1 to 2 grams of psyllium a day mixed with at least 8 ounces of water. If you don't have any intestinal gas or bloating from the psyllium, you can increase the dosage as tolerated. If you are using Metamucil, follow the package directions. If you have an allergic reaction to psyllium, don't use it again.

Get at least 150 minutes per week of activity equivalent in intensity to brisk walking. Many people break that down into 30 minutes of exercise 5 days a week. But whether you get your daily exercise at one time or spread throughout the day is irrelevant to weight loss, says John Jakicic, Ph.D., assistant professor in the department of health, sport, and exercise sciences at the University of

Kansas in Lawrence. So build 10- to 15-minute spurts of activity into your daily routine. Walk to work or get off the bus a couple of blocks from work, and walk up the steps instead of taking the elevator.

Take 400 micrograms of chromium picolinate supplements every day. Chromium makes the insulin in your body work more efficiently, so less is needed to handle the carbohydrates you eat. When your insulin levels are high, fat burning is slowed, more fat is stored, and you gain weight. Chromium supplements may be especially beneficial for people who crave sweets and eat a lot of carbohydrates.

Other Approaches

Cut out what you crave. A food sensitivity can be responsible for your excess pounds by actually making you crave and overeat certain foods, explains Suzanne Myer, R.D., assistant professor and director of dietetics at Bastyr University in Kenmore, Washington. In addition, you could have physical symptoms such as bloating or respiratory problems. Wheat is a common sensitivity, so if you crave bread or cookies, you might have a sensitivity to the wheat in those foods. If you suspect a food sensitivity, cut out the food you crave for 2 weeks and keep track of how you feel, suggests Myer. There is no universal symptom of a food sensitivity, she explains. Whatever your symptom, if you are sensitive to a food, cutting it out should make you feel better. Then introduce the food back into your diet and see how you feel. Often, after cutting the food out for a while and resting your body, you can eat it occasionally with fewer or milder symptoms, she says.

Set a realistic weight-loss goal that is approximately 10 percent of your current weight. When you're trying to lose weight, use the first two digits of your current weight as your weight-loss goal. So if you weigh 200 pounds, your goal is to lose 20 pounds. It is better to reach that small goal and learn to maintain it than to fail to reach an unrealistic goal. If you get discouraged, you are more likely to give up.

Even a 10 percent weight loss has a positive effect on diabetes, high blood pressure, and cholesterol levels, says Gary Foster, Ph.D., clinical director of the weight and eating disorders program at the University of Pennsylvania School of Medicine in Philadelphia. "Losing weight is a tough biological and behavioral challenge. If you can't maintain a 10 percent loss, you won't be able to maintain a 20 percent weight loss because, on average, the less you weigh, the fewer calories you can eat," he says.

As you eat, savor your food's smell. Then take small bites of food and chew well. More odor molecules reach your olfactory bulb, a satiety center in the brain, when you carefully chew your food. Why do this? There is a direct link between your nose and the satiety center in the brain that tells you when you have eaten enough, explains Alan R. Hirsch, neurological director of the Smell and Taste Research Foundation in Chicago and author of *Dr. Hirsch's Guide to Scentsational Weight Loss.* If your satiety center gets enough smells, it sends out signals that you have eaten enough. Eat your food hot, since more natural aromas are released from hot than cold food.

If you have cravings for sweets, especially chocolate, take 300 to 500 milligrams a day of magnesium supplements. Extra magnesium might help manage the cravings, says Dr. Steelman. Note that magnesium is in many multivitamins, so be sure to account for that when deciding on how much more you need to supplement.

Consider a daily supplement of hydroxycitric acid (HCA). It helps decrease the amount of carbohydrates that are stored as fat. Instead, more carbohydrates are stored as glycogen. When the body needs a surge of energy, glycogen is converted to blood sugar, and as glycogen stores increase, appetite decreases. "I have seen it be fairly helpful," says Dr. Steelman. He suggests taking 250 milligrams of HCA three times a day, 30 to 60 minutes before meals. Look for capsules or caplets (such as those from Natrol) that are made from CitriMax, a stable, effective form of hydroxycitric acid.

Add a dash of cayenne pepper, also known as red pepper, or hot-pepper sauce (like Tabasco) to your food several times a day. The active ingredient in hot pepper, capsaicin, stimulates the creation of saliva, salivary amalase (an enzyme involved in the digestion of starch), and hydrochloric acid, all of which improve the digestive process. Moreover, capsaicin may also accelerate metabolism. In research conducted at Oxford Polytechnic Institute in England, dieters who added 1 teaspoon of red-pepper sauce and one teaspoon of mustard to every meal raised their metabolic rates by as much as 25 percent.

Poison Ivy and Poison Oak

The leaves, stems, and roots of poison ivy and poison oak contain an oil called urushiol that triggers an allergic reaction in many people. Your immune system responds to this powerful irritant by attacking it with histamines and other chemicals. The result is red, inflamed, itchy, blistery skin.

The Blended Prescription

Note: To learn about cautions and possible side effects of the remedies in this chapter, see page 253.

Right away, remove and wash your clothes to avoid getting the oil on your skin again. Then wash yourself with soap and water to get the urushiol off your skin. If you act within the first 5 minutes of exposure, you might prevent an outbreak. See your doctor if you develop an itchy rash that is red, swollen, and blistered or involves your face, eyes, hands, or genitals. Here are three options from our blended-medicine experts for a less-itching rash and a faster recovery.

After washing the exposed area, immediately apply these products to the skin. First, apply Tecnu, a lotion containing two patented formulas, to remove the harmful oil from your skin. Tecnu is available at most drugstores. Then use calendula (*Calendula officinalis*) cream or a nonprescription 1 percent hydrocortisone cream to help heal the skin.

Take the homeopathic remedy Rhus tox. 30C. Start with two pellets every 15 minutes for four doses, followed by two pellets every hour on the first day. After that, take two pellets four times a day until the rash goes away.

Run hot water over the affected area. The water should be as hot as you can stand, says Andrew T. Weil, M.D., clinical professor of internal medicine and director of the integrative medicine program at the University of Arizona College of Medicine in Tucson and author of *Spontaneous Healing*. Don't burn yourself with water that is too hot. Running the hot water over the rash briefly intensifies the itching, then makes it stop. As soon as the itching starts again, give your skin the hot-water treatment, which not only provides relief but also reduces the amount of time it takes your skin to heal.

Other Approaches

Soak a washcloth in cold milk and hold it to your skin. Some believe the fats and proteins in the milk soothe the skin, says Mary Ruth Buchness, M.D., chief of dermatology at St. Vincent's Hospital and Medical Center in New York City.

Add a powdered colloidal oatmeal preparation (such as Aveeno) to a tub of water and soak for about 15 minutes. Oatmeal baths are another popular, natural way to soothe the skin.

Prostate Problems

Benign prostatic hyperplasia (BPH) affects more than half the men in the United States over age 50. BPH is an enlargement of the male sex gland known as the prostate—the walnut-size producer of the fluid that carries sperm. The problem is that the prostate encircles the urethra (the tube that carries urine from the bladder). An overinflated prostate constricts the urethra, causing discomfort and urinary problems.

As a result, men with BPH may have the need to urinate frequently, difficulty starting to urinate, weak urine streams, several interruptions in their urine streams that end with a dribble, or a sudden, strong need to urinate. Other disorders, including prostate cancer, can cause some of the same symptoms, but BPH is not cancer and does not increase your chances of developing prostate cancer. Doctors are not entirely sure what causes the prostate to grow as you age, but they think the buildup of the prostate growth hormone dihydrotestosterone may be to blame.

The Blended Prescription

Note: To learn about cautions and possible side effects of the remedies in this chapter, see page 253.

Any man with symptoms of BPH should go to a doctor and undergo a couple of tests—a digital rectal exam of the prostate and a blood test—to make sure that prostate cancer isn't the culprit. The American Cancer Society urges all men to get these tests once a year from the time they are 50 years old, sooner (around age 45) if they have a family history of prostate cancer.

If your doctor determines that you have BPH, there are several herbs and natural supplements that are highly ef-

---

HERBAL POWER

Saw Palmetto

Saw palmetto (*Serenoa repens*) comes from the berry of a dwarf palm tree that grows in the southeastern United States and the Caribbean. Seminole Indians ate saw palmetto seeds to treat urinary problems. Today, it is the most common plant therapy used for benign prostatic hyperplasia (BPH) worldwide.

To relieve the symptoms associated with BPH, take 160 milligrams twice daily of the standardized extract in capsule form, says Mark W. McClure, M.D., a urologist in Raleigh, North Carolina, who practices both alternative and traditional medicine. "It should be standardized to provide 85 to 95 percent of fatty acids and sterols," he adds. Take this dose until symptoms improve, then lower the dose to the lowest amount possible to keep symptoms under control.

Nearly a dozen studies have shown that saw palmetto is effective in the treatment of BPH. Among other things, it decreases the swelling and inflammation of an enlarged prostate. "Saw palmetto can significantly improve your symptoms, and it has fewer side effects and costs less than the drugs that are available," Dr. McClure says.

fective at battling the condition. Here is a five-supplement prescription from our blended-medicine experts that together offers the maximum relief.

Take saw palmetto (*Serenoa repens*), which is one of the most potent and effective natural remedies for BPH. For information on how much of this herbal extract to take and how it affects BPH, see "Herbal Power," opposite.

Take 100 milligrams twice a day of pygeum (*Pygeum africanum*) extract in capsule form. Research has shown that elevated cholesterol levels within the prostate gland are associated with BPH. This herb, extracted from the bark of an African tree, lowers the amount of cholesterol in the prostate and decreases inflammation of the gland. Choose a product standardized to 13 percent total sterols. Take pygeum at this dosage until symptoms improve, then lower the dosage to the lowest possible amount to keep symptoms under control.

Take 120 milligrams twice daily of stinging nettle (*Urtica dioica*) standardized extract in capsule form. The active ingredients in this herb suppress prostatic cell growth and decrease inflammation in the prostate. Take stinging nettle at the recommended dosage until symptoms improve, then lower the dosage to the lowest possible amount to keep symptoms under control. A shopping tip: Look for a formula that contains saw palmetto, pygeum, and stinging nettle. It may be more economical than buying the herbs separately.

Take 30 milligrams a day of zinc picolinate, along with 2 milligrams of copper. Zinc supplements appear effective in shrinking an enlarged prostate. Zinc, however, competes with copper for absorption in your body, which is why you should supplement the two minerals together.

Consider mixing a tablespoon of flaxseed (*Linum usitatissimum*) oil into your food or juice once a day. Essential fatty acids, such as those in flaxseed oil, help prevent inflammation and swelling of the prostate. If you prefer, take the flaxseed oil in supplement form, following the dosage instructions on the package. Flaxseed oil has so many other positive benefits that blended-medicine experts recommend continuous use.

Other Approaches

Stick to a low-fat, high-fiber diet. This helps decrease the cholesterol level within the prostate, protect you from prostate cancer, and prevent obesity, which is associated with BPH, says Mark W. McClure, M.D., a urologist in Raleigh, North Carolina, who practices both alternative and traditional medicine. Strive for a daily intake of 65 grams of fat and 25 grams of fiber. Foods high in fiber include beans, whole-wheat pasta, raspberries, figs, nuts like almonds and peanuts, and dried fruits such as pears, apples, and peaches.

Cut back on meat. Much of the meat sold today contains hormones that are injected into cattle to fatten them up. These hormones may increase the risk for BPH, says Dr. McClure. Even more important, studies show that vegetarians have a lower incidence of prostate cancer compared with meat eaters. If you feel that you must eat meat, buy products whose labels state that no hormone implants were injected into the cattle, he suggests.

Eliminate caffeine from your diet. Caffeine irritates both the bladder and the prostate, worsening the symptoms associated with BPH, says Dr. McClure. "Caffeine stays in your system for 24 hours, so just cutting back won't really help," he says. "You have to completely stop consuming foods and beverages that contain caffeine."

Avoid alcohol and spicy foods. They can irritate your already aggravated bladder and prostate, says Dr. McClure.

Snack on ¼ to ½ cup of pumpkin seeds every day. Pumpkin seeds, which are high in zinc and omega-3 essential fatty acids, have been shown to help relieve the symptoms of BPH. "I recommend eating organic pumpkin seeds, which are free of harmful pesticides," says Dr. McClure. Look for them at health food stores.

Take 1 tablespoon of cod-liver oil daily. Cod-liver oil is rich in omega-3s, which are powerful cancer fighters. "A daily dose of cod-liver oil can lower your risk of developing prostate cancer and may alleviate some of the symptoms of BPH," says Dr. McClure.

SKILLFUL HEALERS

Medical Doctor

If your symptoms include painful urination and a fever, chances are that you have an infection called prostatitis and may need an antibiotic, says Martin K. Gelbard, M.D., clinical professor of urology at the University of California, Los Angeles, School of Medicine; a urologist in Burbank; and author of *Solving Prostate Problems*.

If you indeed have an enlarged prostate, your doctor may prescribe terazosin (Hytrin) or another alpha-blocker designed to relax the muscles around the prostate that are putting pressure on the urethra. "The alpha-blockers are the most rapidly acting medications available for benign prostatic hyperplasia," says Dr. Gelbard. "Your symptoms should improve within a few days of starting on the medication." Another drug often prescribed by doctors is finasteride (Proscar), which actually shrinks the prostate.

Make love to your sweetheart. Ejaculating regularly eases fluid congestion in the prostate and may help relieve urinary symptoms, says Kenneth Goldberg, M.D., founder and director of the Male Health Institute in Irving, Texas.

Psoriasis

In the normal sequence of skin creation, it takes about a month for skin cells to grow, mature, and flake off. But when you have psoriasis, that process is accelerated. New skin can come and go in as little as 3 days. Since your body can't get rid of new skin that quickly, you end up with too much inventory, in the form of white, crusty lesions that usually develop on fast-growth areas like the elbows, knees, scalp, chest, and back. Even your fingernails and toenails grow faster, so they may become discolored, thickened, and separated from the skin.

Psoriasis is not infectious; you can't catch it from someone else. And although it can show up in several family members, it is probably not something you inherit. Emotional stress and infection (like a sore throat) often seem to precede a bout of psoriasis. Further, if your liver doesn't do such a great job filtering out toxins from the bloodstream, psoriasis outbreaks can become even worse.

The Blended Prescription

Note: To learn about cautions and possible side effects of the remedies in this chapter, see page 253.

Since there is no known cure for psoriasis, most natural, alternative, and conventional remedies are aimed at helping to soothe the skin and quell the itching. See your doctor if your psoriasis does not respond to these remedies.

Here is an eight-part blend that addresses the condition on all fronts from our blended-medicine experts.

If possible, expose the affected skin to 15 to 30 minutes of sunlight every day. Ultraviolet light slows down the abnormal growth of skin cells.

Ask your doctor about a prescription for calcipotriene (Dovonex) cream or ointment. Rub it into the lesions twice a day to control the excessive production of skin cells.

Use a 1 percent concentration of hydrocortisone cream (such as Cortizone-10), an over-the-counter formulation, during acute flare-ups. You can apply the cream three times daily. This should provide relief from itching.

Take the following potent mix of skin-healing supplements. If you don't see results after 2 months, discontinue taking these supplements.

Vitamin A: Take 50,000 international units (IU) daily for 2 weeks, then reduce the dose to 10,000 IU

Vitamin E: 400 IU twice a day

Chromium picolinate: 400 micrograms twice a day

Zinc picolinate: 30 milligrams twice a day

Borage (Borago officinalis) *oil:* 1,000 milligrams twice a day

Add a daily tablespoon of flaxseed (*Linum usitatissimum*) oil to food or juice. Also eat cold-water fish such as cod, tuna, or swordfish at least twice a week. If you don't like fish, you can replace it with 2,000 milligrams of fish-oil capsules twice a day. Flaxseed and fish oils have been shown to improve a number of skin conditions, including psoriasis.

Take 200 milligrams of the herb goldenseal (*Hydrastis canadensis*) for 2 weeks, three times a day, then reduce to once a day for a month. Goldenseal contains substances that stop your body from creating polyamines, a chemical linked to psoriasis. Discontinue this treatment if you have no results after 6 weeks.

Twice a day, have 70 milligrams of milk thistle (*Silybum marianum*) capsules. Milk thistle, a popular herb for the liver, also helps combat psoriasis.

Have two pellets, twice a day, of both the homeopathic remedies Arsenicum album 30C and Sulfur 30C. Do this for 2 weeks. Then take two pellets of Petroleum 30C twice daily for 2 more weeks.

Other Approaches

Avoid caffeine and alcohol. Both work to prevent the liver from filtering out toxins, according to Shiva Barton, N.D., a licensed acupuncturist and lead naturopathic physician at the Wellspace Health Center in Cambridge, Massachusetts.

Spray a zinc solution onto affected areas once or twice a day. Zinc solution is available in a spray bottle in health food stores and some drugstores. Daily applications can help stop the itching and heal raw, sore areas faster. Mist your skin with the zinc spray after showering, says Dr. Barton. Reapply about 12 hours later. If you can't find the spray form, make your own by mixing a 150-milligram crushed zinc tablet into 4 ounces of water and pouring the solution into a spray bottle.

Take 50 milligrams of Kaffir potato (*Coleus forskohlii*) capsules two or three times a day. This botanical remedy will help decrease the rate of skin production so that lesions can begin to heal, notes Dr. Barton. Mix the extract with juice or water, and drink.

Rub on chamomile (*Matricaria recutita*) cream as often as you like. Chamomile cream is an anti-inflammatory agent that helps soothe dry, flaky skin. You can continue using it until your skin condition clears up, says Dr. Barton.

Repetitive Stress Injuries

Turn your hand palm up and look at the area where it connects to your wrist. Buried below the surface at that spot is your carpal tunnel—a tight passageway for the tendons and the main nerve that control movement and feeling in your hand. Under normal circumstances, the tendons and nerve easily slide back and forth through the tunnel and everything works fine. But what if you're a little tough on your hands—you spend too many hours pounding the keys on your computer or nailing new shingles on your house or just tightly holding the steering wheel of your car, for example? Then those tendons can swell, pinching the nerve in that tight passageway. The result? In the case of carpal tunnel syndrome, you experience shooting pain in your wrist and forearm, hand numbness, and loss of hand dexterity.

Repetitive stress injuries (RSI) can occur anywhere nerves go through tight passages or tunnels—the feet, ankles, lower legs, shoulders, and neck.

The Blended Prescription

Note: To learn about cautions and possible side effects of the remedies in this chapter, see page 253.

Contact your doctor if you have severe pain, swelling, or any persistent tingling or decreased sensation; tests and supervised therapy may be necessary. If you feel the tired achiness of impending RSI or if you know you have it, use this eight-step prescription from our blended-medicine experts, which mixes common sense with the best of natural supplements.

Spend no more than 4 hours per day—preferably much less—doing the activity that caused the injury. This will relieve the swelling of the tendons, which will lessen the pressure on the nerve, explains Lee Osterman, M.D., professor of orthopedic medicine and hand surgery at Thomas Jefferson University Hospital in Philadelphia and a repetitive-stress-injury specialist at the Philadelphia Hand Clinic.

While doing the activity, take breaks every hour or so. For instance, if hammering aggravates your RSI, break up the time you spend hammering by doing other activities like using a saw, organizing materials, or taking a drink of

---

HERBAL POWER

Red Pepper for Relief

Red pepper, *Capsicum*, cayenne, capsaicin. Different words for the same remedy. Red pepper has six pain-relieving compounds and seven anti-inflammatory agents, says James A. Duke, Ph.D., a botanical consultant, a former ethnobotanist with the U.S. Department of Agriculture who specializes in medicinal plants, and author of *The Green Pharmacy*. Because of these properties, it's great for relieving the achiness and swelling of repetitive stress injuries.

There are a couple of ways you can dose yourself. You can add 3 to 5 teaspoons of powdered cayenne to ¼ cup of skin lotion and rub it on your injured area. Or you can buy a capsaicin-containing salve like Zostrix or Capzacin-P. Apply it as often as needed.

Avoid getting red pepper near your eyes. Also wear rubber gloves and apply just a little cream at a time. "Some people find capsaicin as irritating as the problem they are trying to treat," Dr. Duke cautions.

Dr. Duke also recommends adding red pepper to your diet to stimulate the production of your internal painkillers and reduce your perception of pain.

water, says Dr. Osterman. Break from your activity for 5 to 10 minutes.

Wear a support brace on the affected area while sleeping. There are about 27 different braces available in stores selling medical supplies, notes Dr. Osterman. Pick one that feels comfortable, either with or without a metal support rod in it, and wear it while you sleep. This prevents you from damaging the injured area while resting and speeds healing. Occasionally, you might also want to wear the brace during the aggravating activity, but don't live in it.

Take an over-the-counter anti-inflammatory drug as needed. Nonprescription drugs such as ibuprofen can reduce the swelling of your tendons and the pain that go with RSI. But don't use anti-inflammatories to continue doing the full amount of the activity that caused your injury, warns Dr. Osterman. You could abuse your tendons and nerves to the point where OTC drugs won't help. Instead, use these drugs to help you through particularly trying periods. Always use them as directed on the package, he says.

Take two 375-milligram capsules of bromelain three times a day between meals. Make sure that the supplement has a potency of 2,400 mcu (a standard unit of measurement for enzymes). This enzyme is extracted from pineapples and has powerful anti-inflammatory properties. Bromelain doesn't start working right away, but after a few days, you should start to get relief that is long lasting, says John Collins, N.D., a naturopathic physician and a teacher of homeopathy at the National College of Naturopathic Medicine in Portland, Oregon.

Swallow 50 milligrams of vitamin B$_6$ once a day. Vitamin B$_6$ can help reduce the swelling of the tendons around the nerve and relieve pain. In fact, a deficiency of vitamin B$_6$ is common in people with repetitive stress injuries. If it is helpful, you should begin feeling better in a few weeks and may keep taking the vitamin as a preventive measure.

Take regular doses of St. John's wort. Also known as *Hypericum perforatum*, this herb can soothe the pressured nerves of repetitive stress injuries. You can get it in health food stores; take 300 milligrams a day. In addition to supplements, you can get St. John's wort essential oil and apply it over the affected area as needed for relief.

Consider seeing a chiropractor or an acupuncturist. A chiropractor can adjust the affected area to open the nerve passage, says Irwin Heller, D.C., a chiropractic physician at American WholeHealth Centers in Chicago. Likewise, an acupuncturist can pinpoint spots that will give you considerable relief from pain and swelling.

Other Approaches

Consider taking a homeopathic remedy. Choose one from the following three commonly recommended remedies.

- Hypericum 6C can soothe the pressured nerves of repetitive stress injuries. "This is the first remedy I would try if I had carpal tunnel syndrome," says Stephen Messer, N.D., a naturopathic physician in Eugene, Oregon, and dean of the summer school of the National Center for Homeopathy in Alexandria, Virginia.
- Rhus tox. 6C is great for relieving the stiffness and achiness of repetitive stress injuries. "It's probably the second remedy I would choose," says Dr. Messer.
- Agaricus 6C is good if you have lightninglike shots of pain. It can reduce swelling and pain within hours, notes Dr. Messer.

In all cases, take one pellet three times a day. All of these remedies can be used safely over a long period of time. If you find, however, that they are not working for you after a couple of weeks, stop taking them.

Stretch the injured areas before work and during coffee and lunch breaks. A stretching routine for your whole body is the best preventive measure, says Bob Winkelspecht, an occupational therapist certified in hand therapy at Affinity, an occupational health clinic in Allentown, Pennsylvania. But it is also a good idea to pay particular attention to overused or injured areas. Here are some stretching tips Winkelspecht recommends for the commonly injured wrist and forearm area.

- For fingers, press the lengths of your fingers together, letting them bend at the first knuckles (at the base of the fingers). Your wrists should be somewhat apart, and you should feel the stretch in your fingers.
- For your inside forearms, stretch your arm out straight in front of you, with your palm facing up. Use your other hand to gently bend your fingers down. You should feel the stretch in your inside forearm and wrist. Repeat the process on your other arm.
- For your outside forearm, start with your arm out straight in front of you and your palm facing down. This time, use your other hand to bend your fingers down. While the one hand is pushing down on the fingers, push against the hand with the fingers of your outstretched arm to feel a good stretch along your outside forearm.

Alternate warm- and cold-water compresses. Warm water increases circulation to the area, and cold helps reduce swelling, says Dr. Osterman. So soak a washcloth or towel in warm water and wrap the injured area with it for about 3 minutes. Remove it and apply a cold-water compress for 30 seconds. Repeat the process as often as you like.

Shingles

The first time you got chickenpox, your parents and doctor knew exactly what it was. The second time around, it may be a lot harder to identify. The same herpes zoster virus, lurking in the nerve cells of your spine—often for decades—comes out of hiding to cause shingles, a condition in which parts of your body become inflamed and sore and your skin develops an itchy, red rash and blisters. Often, herpes zoster returns when your immune system is weak from illness, stress, or advanced age.

Shingles often starts with a slight fever, tiredness, or an upset stomach, sometimes with a slight pain on one side of the body. Infected nerves become inflamed and very painful. After a few days, you are likely to get a rash characterized by small, fluid-filled blisters that erupt along the path of the affected nerves. After a week or two, the rash generally subsides and scabs form from the blisters. But the deep-down pain around the nerve can last for months or even years after the skin heals.

The Blended Prescription

Note: To learn about cautions and possible side effects of the remedies in this chapter, see page 253.

If you think you may be developing a case of shingles, see your doctor right away. Unfortunately, there is no way to defend yourself from the virus, but you can help prevent its progress and make yourself somewhat more comfortable. Your doctor can prescribe an antiviral medication such as acyclovir (Zovirax). Since over-the-counter remedies might not be enough to ease the pain, your doctor can also prescribe strong painkillers. After your visit to the doctor, however, there are many other things that you can

HERBAL POWER

Licking It with Licorice

The herb licorice (*Glycyrrhiza glabra*) in its pure form can help fight the herpes zoster virus and reduce the nerve inflammation associated with shingles, says Shiva Barton, N.D., a licensed acupuncturist and lead naturopathic physician at the Wellspace Health Center in Cambridge, Massachusetts. Take 60 drops of licorice tincture three times a day for 3 weeks. If you buy it in capsule form, take 1,000 milligrams three times a day for 3 weeks, he says.

do for yourself, beginning with these five natural steps as suggested by our blended-medicine team.

Take this potent blend of vitamins, amino acid, and herb to help control the condition. Continue with this combination until the lesions clear up.

B-complex vitamin: One tablet of B-complex 50 twice a day

Vitamin C: 2,000 milligrams three times a day

Lysine: 500 milligrams three times a day

Echinacea (Echinacea, *various species*): 200 milligrams four times a day

Cool it with calamine lotion. To soothe itchy skin, pick up calamine lotion at the drugstore and apply it to the affected area not more than four times daily.

Get some homeopathic help. At the onset of shingles, take two pellets of the homeopathic medicine Ranunculus bulboses 6C along with two pellets of Rhus tox. 6C or two pellets of Mezereum 6C every 15 minutes for four doses. Then take two pellets of each every hour for four doses on the first day. After that, take two pellets of each four times a day for an additional week.

Make an oatmeal bath. Stir ½ cup of colloidal oatmeal (like Aveeno) in a tub of cool bathwater and soak in it for 20 to 30 minutes to soothe itching.

See an acupuncturist or a doctor of Chinese medicine for treatment at the first sign of an outbreak of herpes zoster. These forms of healing can be effective in helping to reduce the pain of shingles and speed healing.

Other Approaches

Take 1 tablespoon of black elderberry (*Sambucus nigra*) extract two to four times a day. This herbal extract, an antiviral agent, can reduce nerve inflammation while helping to fight off the herpes zoster virus, says Shiva Barton, N.D., a licensed acupuncturist and lead naturopathic physician at the Wellspace Health Center in Cambridge, Massachusetts. The extract is tasty, but you can also mix it with water or juice, he adds. Stop taking it when your shingles goes away.

Take three or four doses of Arsenicum album 6C a day until the eruptions clear up. If your outbreaks burn worse during the very late hours of the night, shingles is best treated with this homeopathic remedy, according to Sujatha Pillai, a homeopathic physician at American WholeHealth Centers in Chicago. Available in tablet or liquid form, this remedy also helps prevent isolated spots from merging to form larger outbreak areas. If you see improvement in a day or two, keep taking it until your skin is healed.

Rub on some red-pepper cream three or four times a day. Try drugstore creams such as Capzasin-P or Zostrix that contain capsaicin, the active ingredient in red peppers, suggests Dr. Barton. As contrary as it sounds, these "hot" treatments actually relieve the burning that's common after the sores have healed. Don't put this cream on open wounds, however, because it will cause intense, burning pain.

Sinusitis

Parked on both sides of your nose and above your eyes, your sinuses are cavernous pockets that warm and clean air on its way to your lungs. Normally, mucus forms on the surfaces of your sinuses, which are blanketed with tiny hairs called cilia. Each time you inhale, the mucus traps dirt and other airborne debris that the cilia sweep out through tiny drains called ostia. The mucus then rolls down the back of your throat, usually undetected. But when nasal passages clog, thick mucus won't budge, and oxygen levels drop within the nasal cavity. That makes the sinuses perfect breeding grounds for bacteria. The result is inflammation, thick yellow or green mucus, and facial pain—the classic hallmarks of a sinus infection, or sinusitis.

The Blended Prescription

Note: To learn about cautions and possible side effects of the remedies in this chapter, see page 253.

To clear up sinusitis, you must kill the infection as well as clear out the blockages. First, see your doctor if you have the signs of sinusitis, especially if your symptoms last more than 3 days or if you develop a fever or severe pain around your sinuses. If you have a bacterial infection, you will probably need an antibiotic. In addition, here is a three-step prescription from our blended-medicine experts for quick and effective relief.

SKILLFUL HEALERS

Acupuncture

If you really want fast relief from a nagging sinus infection, consider a visit to an acupuncturist. A 25- to 30-minute treatment can clear your head, reduce pain and inflammation, and relieve pressure immediately, says Tony Lu, M.D., an integrative medicine specialist and licensed acupuncturist at American WholeHealth Centers in Chicago. "I use acupuncture for immediate relief because antibiotics may not start working for several days. Acupuncture starts the draining process right away, and it enhances your immune system so the body can battle the infection," he says.

During your visit, your acupuncturist may insert needles in your upper back to strengthen your immune system. Needles may be placed on both sides of your nose and in parts of your hands, arms, and legs to stimulate blood flow and white blood cell activity to the nasal area and help to reduce inflammation in the mucous membranes, says Dr. Lu.

To loosen up mucus, inhale steam. Here's the best approach: Add ¼ teaspoon of Vicks VapoRub or five drops of eucalyptus (*Eucalyptus globulus*) essential oil to a pan of water. Heat it until boiling, then remove from the stove. Drape a towel over your head and lean over the pan. Keeping your head at least 6 inches away from the water, inhale the steam through both nostrils. Hold this position for 5 to 10 minutes, or until the water cools down. Blow your nose frequently while inhaling the steam. Do this every few hours, if possible.

Use an over-the-counter nasal decongestant spray to open sinus passages so mucus can flow more easily. You can try sprays such as Afrin. Follow the package instructions, but use the spray no more than 4 days.

Several herbs and vitamins are effective in the battle against sinusitis. Here are a few that you can take concurrently for absolute maximum healing effect.

Echinacea (Echinacea purpurea): Take 200 milligrams of this herb five times a day for 5 days. Echinacea is full of antiviral properties, and it serves as a stimulant to the immune system, says Kristy Fassler, N.D., a naturopathic physician in Portsmouth, New Hampshire.

Goldenseal root (Hydrastis canadensis): Take 200 milligrams five times a day for 5 days. Goldenseal root fights infection and helps control mucus, Dr. Fassler explains.

Vitamin A: Take 50,000 international units (IU) per day. Vitamin A is known as the anti-infection vitamin.

Bromelain: Take a 375-milligram capsule at a potency of 2,400 mcu (a standard unit of measurement for enzymes) up to three times a day between meals for 5 days. Bromelain, an enzyme found in pineapple, breaks up and dries mucus very effectively, Dr. Fassler explains.

Other Approaches

Try a position that gives you relief. Lie on your back, with your buttocks pushed against the base of a wall and your legs raised together against the wall, suggests Larry Payne, Ph.D., director of the Samata Yoga Center in Los Angeles and chairman of the International Association of Yoga Therapists. Hold this position for 7 to 15 minutes, he advises. "This changes bloodflow within the body and changes the flow of your body's lymphatic fluids—the fluids that flow from the space between the body cells into the bloodstream. For the first few minutes, pressure in your sinuses will increase. But after a while, the mucus in your sinuses starts loosening."

Don't do this exercise if you have high blood pressure, stroke risk, or glaucoma, Dr. Payne cautions.

Sore Throat

Like a magnet, the throat attracts viruses and other airborne irritants that cling to its delicate tissues. Usually, your body finds a way to quickly eradicate the irritant. But when conditions are right, the invader settles in and reproduces. That sparks a stronger response from the immune system that includes bombarding the invading colony with chemicals and white blood cells. These chemicals—and the toxins produced by viruses—are what cause the telltale burning sensation and inflammation of a sore throat. Other mischief makers are smoking, dry air, environmental pollution, bacterial infections, and stomach acid reflux.

The Blended Prescription

Note: To learn about cautions and possible side effects of the remedies in this chapter, see page 253.

You should always see a doctor if your sore throat is accompanied by a rash, earache, discolored mucus, pus-covered tonsils, a high temperature (over 100°F), chest pain, or shortness of breath. Otherwise, you can pretty much treat your sore throat on your own. When you have a cold or flu along with a sore throat, you will want a combination of remedies, so be sure to see the prescriptions in this book for colds and flu as well as the ones here. These seven remedies recommended by our blended-medicine experts reduce pain and inflammation, strengthen your immune system, and shorten the duration of the sore throat.

Take up to 1,000 milligrams of acetaminophen every 4 hours. This will help relieve throat pain.

Gargle frequently. Use warm water and add 40 drops of echinacea (*Echinacea purpurea*) tincture or simply a little salt to soothe your sore throat.

HERBAL POWER

Some Real Hip Tea

Rose hip tea will make your sore throat feel much better, says Ellen Evert Hopman, a master herbalist in Amherst, Massachusetts; a professional member of the American Herbalists Guild; and author of *Tree Medicine, Tree Magic*. The vitamin C in the rose hips is quickly absorbed by the body to help battle invading viruses, she says.

Place 2 tablespoons of rose hips into a non-aluminum pot. Add 1 cup of water. Cover the pot tightly and let simmer for 20 to 30 minutes. Strain the tea into a cup through a coffee filter and add freshly squeezed lemon juice and honey to taste. "Drink it at a very warm but comfortable temperature," advises Hopman.

You can also put 20 to 90 drops of echinacea (*Echinacea purpurea*) tincture in the tea to give your immune system that extra "oomph" it needs to fight the infection.

Take two 375-milligram capsules of bromelain three times a day between meals until symptoms are relieved. Make sure that the supplement has a potency of 2,400 mcu (a standard unit of measurement for enzymes). Bromelain is an enzyme abundant in fresh pineapple but also available as a supplement that is believed to improve circulation and treat inflammation as well as improve the effects of some antibiotics.

Three times a day for 5 days, take 50,000 international units (IU) of beta-carotene and 2,000 milligrams of vitamin C. Also take 400 IU of vitamin E twice a day for up to 5 days. Each of these vitamins bolsters the immune system.

Take a 15-milligram zinc gluconate lozenge (such as Cold-Eeze) every 2 to 3 hours as needed. For maximum effectiveness, make sure that you suck on the lozenge until it completely dissolves in your mouth.

For herbal remedies, take 200 milligrams of any of the following immune-stimulating herbs four times a day for up to 5 days. Try echinacea (*Echinacea purpurea*), goldenseal (*Hydrastis canadensis*), or astragalus (*Astragalus membranaceus*).

Have a homeopathic dose of Belladonna 6C, Lachesis 6C, or Lycopodium 6C. Take two pellets every 15 minutes for four doses, then two pellets every hour for four doses. After that, take two pellets every 6 hours until your symptoms are gone.

Other Approaches

Gargle with a sage-eucalyptus tea. Boil 8 ounces of water, add 2 teaspoons each of dried sage (*Salvia officinalis*) and eucalyptus (*Eucalyptus globulus*) leaves, and let steep for 20 to 30 minutes. Let the tea cool, strain, then gargle with it throughout the day as needed, says Ellen Evert Hopman, a master herbalist in Amherst, Massachusetts; a professional member of the American Herbalists Guild; and author of *Tree Medicine*, *Tree Magic*. Sage and eucalyptus have antibacterial properties to help heal your sore throat; sage is also an antiviral and anti-inflammatory.

Treat yourself to soothing supplements. Take 3,000 milligrams of vitamin C, 400 IU of vitamin E, 25,000 milligrams of beta-carotene, 50 micrograms of selenium, and 500 milligrams of mixed bioflavonoids daily until symptoms go away, recommends Keith Berndtson, M.D., an integrative medicine specialist at American WholeHealth Centers in Chicago. These vitamins and minerals have antiviral and antibacterial compounds and rev up your immune system, he says.

Sunburn

Sunburn is pretty straightforward: If you stay in the sun too long, you get burned. With a mild sunburn, the sun's ultraviolet radiation singes the cells in the first layer of your skin, the epidermis. But a more severe sunburn can damage the second layer of skin, called the dermis, home of hair follicles and living nerves. When the dermis is burned, blood vessels there might spill toxins into the inflamed area, causing the skin layers to swell so much that they actually separate, creating a blister.

The Blended Prescription

Note: To learn about cautions and possible side effects of the remedies in this chapter, see page 253.

If you get badly sunburned and blistered and experience chills, fever, or nausea, seek professional care immediately. These symptoms indicate a serious condition such as sun poisoning. But if your burn is mild, here are seven ways to make amends to your skin for those sizzling hours of outdoor fun, according to our blended-medicine experts.

Break the end of a leaf from an aloe vera plant and squeeze the clear gel inside directly on the burn. Where to find a plant? If you are smart, in your home. Aloe vera is an attractive and hard-to-kill houseplant whose gel is useful for a number of skin problems. Don't have access to the real thing? Then buy a gel or lotion that contains mostly aloe vera, and spread it on your skin to ease the pain as needed.

Pick up some calendula (*Calendula officinalis*) cream to reduce inflammation and begin the healing. Use it along with aloe vera as directed and needed.

Soak a washcloth in witch hazel or cold milk. Wring it out and press it on the damaged skin for a cooling effect. Repeat the process whenever the washcloth warms up.

Put 1 cup of baking soda in lukewarm bathwater and soak in it for about 30 minutes. Baking soda is an effective remedy for soothing the skin.

Apply a nonprescription 1 percent hydrocortisone cream. A hydrocortisone cream (like Cortizone-10) can reduce itching. Use it no more than three times daily.

Take vitamins C and E. To bring down sunburn swelling, take 1,000 milligrams of vitamin C twice a day. And to speed healing, take 400 international units (IU) of vitamin E twice a day.

Once a day, add 2 teaspoons of flaxseed (*Linum usitatissimum*) oil to food or juice. Flaxseed can help protect damaged or inflamed tissue.

Taste and Smell Problems

When you stop to smell the roses or savor your favorite meal, odor-carrying molecules travel up your nose and connect with smell-receptor nerves. These receptors (called olfactory nerves) carry smell messages to your brain, where they are processed and translated into sweet aromas and scrumptious flavors.

This delicate process doesn't always run smoothly, however. Nasal polyps and congestion from a cold, allergy, or sinus infection can cause temporary smell and taste loss. An accidental blow to your head can sever your olfactory nerves. A vitamin or mineral deficiency, certain prescription drugs, and environmental toxins can dull your senses. So can alcohol. Aging, too, gradually impairs smell and taste. At 80, your nose will work about half as well as it did when you were 30.

The Blended Prescription

Note: To learn about cautions and possible side effects of the remedies in this chapter, see page 253.

If your taste and smell problems last for more than 3 months, you should see a doctor. Problems with these senses, in some cases, can indicate a serious condition such as cancer or thyroid problems. But in most cases, you can treat taste and smell problems on your own. Here is a four-step prescription from our panel of blended-medicine experts for recovering your enjoyment of scents and flavors.

Add Tabasco and other spicy seasonings to your food. They help wake up your tastebuds.

Fill up on seafood for extra zinc. Scientists have found that a deficiency of zinc can impair your senses of smell and taste. To make up for a shortfall, you need at least 30 milligrams of zinc a day. You can get that—and more—

through your diet: Just six steamed oysters pack more than 76 milligrams of zinc. Or if you prefer, supplement your diet with 30 milligrams of zinc picolinate and 2 milligrams of copper, taken twice a day, for at least a 3-month trial. Note that zinc competes with copper for absorption in your body, which is why you should supplement the two minerals together.

Have a B-complex 50 vitamin twice a day along with one additional 50-milligram vitamin B_6 tablet. B vitamins help keep the body's nervous system, including the parts that govern taste and smell, at optimum levels.

Put a 1,000-microgram vitamin B_{12} tablet containing 1 milligram of folic acid under your tongue and let it dissolve. Do this once every day. Vitamin B_{12} and folic acid are usually sold together in tablet form. Because of B_{12}'s important nerve-protecting function, it may help with taste and smell problems.

Other Approaches

Eat antioxidant-rich foods in addition to taking super-charged antioxidants. Take 500 milligrams of mixed bioflavonoids along with these specific bioflavonoids: 100 milligrams of hesperidin, 25 milligrams of rutin, and 100 milligrams of quercetin a day, says Keith Berndtson, M.D., an integrative medicine specialist at American Whole-Health Centers in Chicago. And don't forget that fruits and vegetables are great sources of antioxidant compounds, he says. You can't eat enough fruits and vegetables to make a real difference in your taste and smell receptors; you will still need supplementation. But it is always good to get antioxidants from food as well as through supplements, he says.

If chronic sinusitis is hampering your sense of smell, apply some pressure. Place the palm of each hand on your forehead. Turn each hand slightly outward so that the sides of your hands are touching the center of your forehead, with your thumbs facing outward. Firmly press the side of each hand into your forehead, then, continuing the pressure, sweep your hands across to the outer edges. Repeat as often as needed to clear sinus passages, suggests Alan Uretz, an acupuncturist and traditional Chinese medicine physician at American WholeHealth Centers in Chicago.

To clear the lower sinus area, place the outer edge of each hand on each side of your nose. Press firmly and sweep your hands across your sinus area toward the outer edges of your cheekbones. "This will open up your sinuses and stimulate your sense of smell and taste," Uretz says.

Consider visiting an acupuncturist. With acupuncture, it is possible to stimulate neural transmitters in the brain that are associated with smell, says Tony Lu, M.D., an integrative medicine specialist and licensed acupuncturist at American WholeHealth Centers in Chicago.

During treatment, the acupuncturist may insert needles in a series of points in your legs and arms. The objective is to stimulate what is called the intracerebral circulation meridian. "This stimulates circulation and attracts nutrients to the olfactory nerve area and the brain," says Dr. Lu.

Temporomandibular Disorder

If you have temporomandibular disorder, your upper and lower jaws have somehow become misaligned, putting stress on the pair of hinges that work your jawbone. This misalignment can be due to a head injury, bad dental work, or missing teeth. More likely, you just have a lot of muscle tension, and you unconsciously clench and grind your teeth. Although the problem is basically in the joints, temporomandibular disorder (TMD) can set off a range of symptoms including earaches, headaches,

SKILLFUL HEALERS

Biofeedback

If your temporomandibular disorder is stress-related, biofeedback could be your best bet to alleviate the ache associated with it. In biofeedback, you are hooked up to a machine that measures muscle tension. Painless electrodes are placed on your jaw joints and sometimes on your forehead. "The muscles of the face and head are very integrated," explains Cary Rothstein, Ph.D., a psychologist and director of biofeedback services at Crossroads Center for Psychiatry and Psychology in Doylestown, Pennsylvania. "If you ask someone to clench his teeth, you will see the forehead muscles respond as well as muscles in the jaw."

Once you are hooked up, the biofeedback therapist may ask you to consciously relax your jaw muscles. Or you may be put through a little stress test to become aware of unconscious clenching. "This allows you to see what you actually do with your jaw and face muscles," says Dr. Rothstein.

Along with weekly or biweekly biofeedback sessions, you likely will be asked to practice some relaxation techniques at home. Dr. Rothstein gives his patients an audiotape to listen to daily as part of treatment. "The equipment helps you gain control of the muscles, but you need to learn to cope with stress as well," he observes.

toothaches, and facial pain. Or you might find that those joints click or grind every time you open and close your mouth.

The Blended Prescription

Note: To learn about cautions and possible side effects of the remedies in this chapter, see page 253.

Sometimes people with TMD pain start to get over it as soon as they learn ways to reduce stress and keep the jaw area relaxed. It is a good idea, however, to see a doctor to rule out other diseases if you have the symptoms mentioned above. But when jaw-joint pain has set in and you know it is from TMD, follow this four-step prescription from our blended-medicine experts.

Alternate between cold and warm compresses on the jaw joints. The cold compress helps relieve the pain; the warm compress reduces inflammation. Place the compress right over the affected joint, which is usually slightly below and in front of your ears (feel around while opening and closing your mouth to get the correct location). Rotate warm and cold compresses for 10 to 15 minutes each, three or four times a day, until the pain subsides. To keep the warm compress from cooling, periodically run it under comfortably warm water during the process.

Take an over-the-counter pain reliever as instructed on the bottle. Acetaminophen will ease the hurt, while aspirin or ibuprofen will help reduce inflammation as well as relieve the pain. The latter two, however, are hard on your stomach.

Eat a soft or liquid diet for a few days to minimize work for your jawbone. The rest helps it heal more quickly.

If pain persists, consider seeing an alternative-healing practitioner. Examples of healing practices that are effective in treating TMD include acupressure, chiropractic, acupuncture, and cranial-sacral therapeutic massage.

Other Approaches

Whether you are sitting or standing, make sure that your ears, shoulders, and hips are in line. If you walk around with your chin jutting out, shoulders hunched, and neck craned forward, you are contributing to TMD trouble, says Bernadette Jaeger, D.D.S., associate professor of diagnostic sciences and orofacial pain at the University of California, Los Angeles, School of Dentistry.

Make your jaws work a little easier by getting your posture in line on a regular basis, checking every 2 hours or even more often if you are really stressed or feeling a lot of pain. To adjust your posture, Dr. Jaeger advises that you move your shoulders backward, relax them down, then lift your chest while you let your knees relax. Finally, move your head back so that your ears are in line with your shoulders. Whenever you are standing, lean forward slightly so that your weight falls on the balls of your feet. Your head will then move back and into alignment automatically.

Put your tongue in its proper place. If you habitually clench or grind your teeth, you can learn a tongue-placement trick for keeping jaw muscles loose instead of locked.

Make the sound of the letter N, placing your tongue on the roof of your mouth just behind your upper front teeth. This position keeps your upper and lower jaws slightly separated and the muscles relaxed even if your lips happen to be closed, says Dr. Jaeger. Try to remind yourself to return to the "N" position every couple of hours as well as after eating or having a conversation.

Tendinitis

Tendons are strong, white, fibrous tissues that connect muscles to bones. (One of the most famous tendons is the Achilles, which connects your heel bone to your calf muscle.) Overuse, injury, disease, and even calcium deposits can cause a tendon to become inflamed. When that happens, it presses on nerves and other tissue and generally causes a tremendous amount of pain. At or around the joint, you might experience tenderness, numbness or tingling, low-grade swelling, and stiffness that can make movement painful. Tendinitis usually crops up in shoulders, wrists, heels, and elbows.

The Blended Prescription

Note: To learn about cautions and possible side effects of the remedies in this chapter, see page 253.

If your pain is severe or your movement severely restricted, it is a good idea to check with your doctor. If you have had an injury and are uncertain of the extent of damage caused, see your doctor for a proper diagnosis.

If you mix up the right brew of remedies, tendinitis can heal in about 2 weeks. Here are four important healing steps as prescribed by our blended-medicine experts.

Start with the primary treatment for muscle injuries, a healing system denoted by the acronym RICE. Here is how to do it.

Rest. When tendinitis strikes, immediately stop what you are doing and rest the afflicted joint. It is often tough to do, but staying away from activities that hurt is an expressway to healing, says Steven Subotnick, D.P.M., N.D., Ph.D., clinical professor of biomechanics and surgery at the California College of Podiatric Medicine in Hayward, a specialist in sports medicine, and author of *Sports and Exercise Injuries*. Don't return to an activity until it doesn't hurt to do it.

Ice. As soon as you can, ice the joint for 20 minutes. Repeat every 6 to 8 hours or until the pain and swelling go down. Specially purchased ice packs, a plastic bag filled with ice cubes, or a bag of frozen vegetables works, says Dr. Subotnick. To be safe, wrap whatever ice pack you use in a towel.

Compress. After icing, wrap the joint with an elastic bandage. "The wrap helps provide heat, restricts motion, and works to 'pump out' swelling," says Dale Anderson, M.D., clinical assistant professor at the University of Minnesota Medical School in Minneapolis and author of *Muscle Pain Relief in 90 Seconds: The Fold and Hold Method*. To make sure the bandage isn't on too tight, check your circulation every 15 minutes or so by squeezing a point on your body below the bandaged injury. It should return to its normal color when you release. If it remains white, loosen the bandage immediately.

Elevate. Finally, keep the inflamed tendon and joint elevated as much as you can. If it's your knee or ankle with tendinitis, keep it above your hip. If it's your elbow, wrist, or shoulder, keep it above your heart (that might mean propping it up in bed with pillows). Elevation helps keep the joint from swelling more. Try to keep the injured area elevated for at least 20 minutes, three or four times a day.

Take an anti-inflammatory over-the-counter drug such as ibuprofen for no more than 10 days at a time. Dose yourself according to the directions on the bottle. If you want a natural alternative, try bromelain supplements. Bromelain is an enzyme extracted from pineapple that works as an anti-inflammatory. Take two 375-milligram capsules at a potency of 2,400 mcu (a standard unit of measurement for enzymes) three times a day between meals.

Apply arnica (*Arnica montana*) ointment or Triflora Gel over the painful areas every 2 to 3 hours. These herbal ointments provide relief from pain and swelling. Arnica is derived from the arnica flower; Triflora contains wild rosemary, comfrey, and a very dilute form of poison ivy. Both are available at health food stores.

In addition, take a homeopathic remedy for pain relief, reduced swelling, and less tenderness. There are four to choose from: Arnica 6C, Rhus tox. 6C, Ruta graveolens 6C, and Bryonia 6C. The dosage should be the same no matter which one you pick: two pellets every 15 minutes (up to 10 doses) until discomfort lessens, then two pellets every 4 hours until the pain is completely gone. The remedies can be switched if they don't seem to be working.

Other Approaches

Practice the Fold and Hold technique for 90 seconds, three times a day, for 3 days straight. The Fold and Hold method helps relax and relieve tension from the muscles surrounding the area where you have tendinitis, says Dr. Anderson.

Use your finger to find the exact point on your body that is tender. If you are working on your shoulder, for example, that tender spot could be hidden under one of the many bones around your shoulder, or it could be in the deep, thick muscles along the back of your shoulder.

Next, move your body to "fold" the area into a position that makes the tender spot feel better. With the shoulder as an example again, raising your arm above your head is often the most comfortable position. You could lie down or lean against a wall on the raised-arm side of your body.

This pushes your shoulder farther toward the center of your body, says Dr. Anderson. You can either keep your finger on the tender spot or remove it.

Hold that position for at least 90 seconds, then gently and slowly return to a normal position.

Take 2,000 milligrams of ginger (*Zingiber officinale*) three times a day. Ginger is a powerful anti-inflammatory that works best when used with bromelain, says John Collins, N.D., a naturopathic physician and a teacher of homeopathy at the National College of Naturopathic Medicine in Portland, Oregon. You can buy both at health food stores. Take them until the tendinitis goes away.

Smooth some red-pepper cream on your tendinitis three or four times a day. Red pepper (*Capsicum*, various species) helps knock the pain right out of your tendinitis. It removes the substance that's responsible for transmitting pain signals through the nerves, says Dr. Collins. You can buy it in ointment or cream form from health food stores. Be careful not to get it in or near your eyes. Also, test your red-pepper cream on a small amount of skin first. If the skin becomes irritated, discontinue use.

Spread on Traumed, a homeopathic topical cream, four or five times a day. Traumed is very useful for reducing pain, swelling, and tenderness, Dr. Subotnick says. This cream is available at health food stores.

Take 2,000 to 3,000 milligrams of vitamin C two or three times a day. Vitamin C helps with structural healing, notes Dr. Collins. Take this amount of vitamin C for the first 1 to 2 weeks of your tendinitis.

Take 1,000 milligrams of mixed bioflavonoids for as long as you have tendinitis pain, plus a few days more. Bioflavonoids work well with vitamin C to reduce swelling and pain, says Dr. Collins. It is important to continue taking them for a few days after your pain has resolved in order to prevent a relapse, he says. You can buy them in most health food stores. Among the bioflavonoids you might see listed on the bottle are grapeseed extract and pine bark extract. Bioflavonoids don't start working right away, but they are very effective at reducing pain and swelling, he says.

Use 400 to 600 milligrams of turmeric (*Curcuma longa*) three times a day. Turmeric is effective in relieving the inflammation of tendinitis. Best of all, this spice, which is available in capsule form, may help protect the stomach lining from ulcer formation and against damage done by anti-inflammatory agents, says Dr. Collins. You can buy the capsules in health food stores.

Toothache

It can be ice-cold water, a hard piece of popcorn, or an elbow to the molars. But whatever the cause of the toothache, you can be sure that a sleeping nerve ending has been startled into agony. Sometimes, that exposed nerve is being frayed by an encroaching cavity. Or perhaps you have receding gums that expose sensitive nerve endings to heat and cold. A tooth might be cracked or chipped—or food might be caught between your teeth, creating pressure and gum irritation.

The Blended Prescription

Note: To learn about cautions and possible side effects of the remedies in this chapter, see page 253.

When toothache strikes, you can use some persuasive techniques to halt the immediate pain, but you need to call your dentist for the earliest available appointment to get to the root of the problem. There are some things—toothaches being one of them—that you just can't fix at home. Meanwhile, here is a five-step prescription from our blended-medicine experts for dulling the pain and helping the healing.

Apply a cold compress to the painful spot. You can use a store-bought compress, a bag of frozen vegetables, or a plastic bag of ice; wrap the pack in a towel. Leave it on for no more than 20 minutes at a time. The cold helps to relieve the pain and reduce any swelling.

Take an over-the-counter pain reliever for quick and effective relief. Painkillers made with acetaminophen are the safest for your body, but they don't help with swelling. Aspirin and ibuprofen both kill pain and reduce inflammation, but they are harder on your system and wouldn't be appropriate if your gums are prone to bleeding. Take the pain reliever according to package directions.

Take flavonoid and folic acid supplements to reduce gum inflammation. For a flavonoid, you can take 50 to 100 milligrams of grapeseed extract three times a day or 500 to 1,000 milligrams of citrus bioflavonoids three times a day. For folic acid, take 2 milligrams (2,000 micrograms) daily until the toothache passes.

If your teeth or gums are usually sensitive to the cold, use a special toothpaste for sensitive teeth. These toothpastes contain a desensitizing agent that forms a protective layer on the tooth or exposed gum tissue, says Meena Shah, D.D.S., a dentist in Lake Grove, New York. Look for brands like Sensodyne and Sensitivity Protection Crest. But you should still tell your dentist about the pain you are experiencing, notes Dr. Shah.

If you suspect that a sinus condition or a dental abscess is causing the pain, take two potent herbs. Take 300 milligrams of both goldenseal (*Hydrastis canadensis*) and echinacea (*Echinacea purpurea*) in capsule form three times a day for 1 week. These herbs may offer some antibacterial and antiviral protection.

Other Approaches

Dab some dilute clove oil on your throbbing tooth. Clove (*Syzygium aromaticum*) oil has anesthetic and antiseptic properties. But don't swallow the oil. Mix it with a small amount of almond oil, then place it directly on the tooth or on the sore gum until the throbbing pain is gone, suggests James A. Duke, Ph.D., a botanical consultant, a former ethnobotanist with the U.S. Department of Agriculture who specializes in medicinal plants, and author of *The Green Pharmacy*. You can buy over-the-counter preparations of clove oil.

If you have lost a filling, use a piece of cotton dipped in clove oil as a temporary pain stopper. Roll the material into a pellet and place it in the tooth as a homemade temporary filling, suggests Dr. Shah. This is only an emergency measure, but it will tide you over until you can get to your dentist and have the tooth filled.

Stimulate an acupressure point between your thumb and forefinger to get quick relief. Work on the hand that's on the opposite side of your body from the toothache, says Ken Hiser, a certified shiatsu practitioner and tai chi instructor in Reading, Pennsylvania. You need to find the tender spot between the webbing of your thumb and forefinger. To find this acupressure point, squeeze around in that area with the opposite thumb and forefinger until you feel a tenderness. Continue to squeeze that spot firmly, moving the pressure in a circular motion until the toothache eases. You can return to the spot and apply more pressure every 10 minutes, if needed.

If your tooth gets a hard knock, take Arnica right away. This homeopathic remedy is the right choice if you have a toothache from some kind of direct impact, like a run-in with a doorjamb, says Michael Lipelt, N.D., D.D.S., a naturopathic physician, biological dentist, and licensed acupuncturist at Stillpoint Family Health Services in Sebastopol, California. Take one dose of Arnica in 12X or 30X potency every 15 to 20 minutes until you feel better.

If food is stuck between your teeth, rinse with lukewarm water, then floss. "You may want to try one of the new shred-proof flosses if you have very tight contact between your teeth," says Dr. Shah. Remember that stuck food can lead to a toothache, so keep your choppers clean.

Ulcers

Although many people think that stress causes stomach ulcers, scientists have discovered that in most cases the real culprits are burrowing, spiral-shaped bacteria known as *Helicobacter pylori*. How these bacteria wiggle their way into your stomach lining is unclear, but medical experts believe that contaminated food or water may be to blame. Once in your body, the *H. pylori* dig their way into your stomach's protective mucous lining and secrete an enzyme that shields them from stomach acid.

The bacteria's burrowing can cause a sore that can turn into a small hole if it is left untreated. As stomach acid hits the sore, you may feel a burning, gnawing, and aching in your abdominal area. Worse yet, you might discover blood in your feces if an ulcer has eaten away a sufficient portion of your stomach lining to cause blood to leak into your stomach.

The Blended Prescription

Note: To learn about cautions and possible side effects of the remedies in this chapter, see page 253.

This is one medical problem that can be easily diagnosed with conventional medicine. Tests exist—and better ones are on the way—to quickly determine whether *H. pylori* have taken residence inside your stomach. If the answer is yes, a combination of antibiotics should kill the bacteria and end the ulcers. All this presupposes a visit to your doctor. So if ulcer pain hits, make an appointment.

That said, there is much you can do on your own to minimize the hurt and spread of ulcers and to maximize the healing once the bacteria are ousted. Here is a seven-step prescription for exactly that, as prescribed by our blended-medicine experts.

Use antacids such as Maalox, Tums, or Mylanta, following the instructions on the package. There is a good reason why antacids are among the best-selling medications in the United States: They do a great job of immediately neutralizing acid that has pooled up in your digestive tract and that likely is gnawing painfully at your ulcer. They differ in the mineral they use to neutralize the acid, but all are effective. Making a choice comes down to how well each medication works for you.

When ulcer pain hits, take histamine receptor blockers, following the package directions, to prevent more acid from being made. Until the discovery of *H. pylori*, H_2 blockers were the drugs of choice for treating ulcers. These medicines reduce stomach acid secretion by as much as 80 percent. Once available only by prescription, many are sold over the counter (though in a somewhat weaker form). There are four types of H_2 blockers, but all work well. Popular brands include Zantac, Tagamet, and Pepcid-AC. If you take antacids as well as H_2 blockers, take them at least 2 hours apart to make sure the antacid does not hinder the absorption of the H_2 blockers.

Avoid milk and other dairy products. If you are having a bout of ulcers or are prone to them because of a weakened immune system, it is best to steer clear of these products. They can increase stomach acid.

Avoid excessive alcohol, caffeine, and smoking. These vices can cause ulcers independent of the *H. pylori* bacteria, mainly by increasing stomach acid production.

Take some acetaminophen when pain strikes. Aspirin, ibuprofen, and other painkillers that collectively are known as nonsteroidal anti-inflammatory drugs (NSAIDs) have been shown to cause ulcers when taken in excess. So when pain hits your body and you don't need anti-inflammatory medicine—headaches are a good example—opt for acetaminophen.

Eat a high-fiber diet (at least 20 to 25 grams every day) to reduce the recurrence rate of ulcers. Fibrous foods help

---

HERBAL POWER

A Healing Combo

Two ulcer-calming herbs, slippery elm (*Ulmus rubra*) and goldenseal (*Hydrastis canadensis*), combine to make a powerful healing team, says Mark Stengler, N.D., a naturopathic physician in Carlsbad, California, and author of *The Natural Physician*.

He recommends taking one 500-milligram capsule of slippery elm or 30 drops of its tincture dissolved in ¼ cup of warm water three times daily (let it stand for a few minutes for the alcohol to evaporate—that will improve the taste). For goldenseal, take two 500-milligram capsules three times a day. These herbs coat and soothe the stomach lining.

absorb acid and keep the digestive tract clean and healthy. Eat more cereals, whole-grain breads, pasta, beans, and vegetables to get the fiber you need.

Take two 500-milligram tablets of deglycyrrhizinated licorice (DGL) and allow them to dissolve slowly in your mouth ½ hour before meals. Or take ½ teaspoon of DGL powder and let that slowly dissolve in your mouth for the same effect. This natural product protects and heals your stomach lining in a soothing way, says Andrew T. Weil, M.D., clinical professor of internal medicine and director of the integrative medicine program at the University of Arizona College of Medicine in Tucson and author of *Spontaneous Healing*.

As an alternative, you can take 30 drops of DGL tincture dissolved in warm water three times a day for the same result, says Mark Stengler, N.D., a naturopathic physician in Carlsbad, California, and author of *The Natural Physician*.

Other Approaches

Sip lukewarm chamomile (*Matricaria recutita*) tea three times a day. For best results, drink this herbal tea on an empty stomach, says Dr. Stengler. Or take one capsule or 30 drops of chamomile tincture dissolved in ¼ cup of warm water for the same results, he suggests. Chamomile contains azulene, a potent anti-inflammatory agent that may help heal ulcers.

During periods of stomach distress, eat warmed soft foods, such as steamed white rice and steamed zucchini, and warm vegetable, cabbage, or miso soup. These kinds of foods are easier to digest, explains David J. Nickel, O.M.D., a doctor of Oriental medicine and licensed acupuncturist in Santa Monica, California. Avoid eating raw foods like nuts, granola, and uncooked carrots. "Anything uncooked, in general, is more difficult to digest, especially if your stomach lining is irritated," he says.

Take 200 milligrams of cat's claw (*Uncaria tomentosa*) three times a day. This herb eliminates infections in the gastrointestinal tract as it helps heal your stomach lining, says Dr. Stengler.

Take two doses a day of Nux vomica 30C. This homeopathic remedy is most commonly used for neutralizing excess stomach acid and offering fast relief from ulcer pain, according to Dr. Stengler.

Fight ulcers with vitamins A, B-complex, and E. These three vitamins, in combination, repair the gastrointestinal tract, fight inflammation, and heal the stomach, says Dr. Stengler. He recommends taking a daily dose of 50,000 international units (IU) of vitamin A, 50 milligrams of vitamin B-complex, and 800 IU of vitamin E for best results.

Sprinkle cayenne pepper into your favorite spicy dish. This red pepper acts as a natural anesthetic and brings blood to the surface of the tissue, says Dr. Weil. You can even take it as a tea—with ¼ teaspoon of cayenne pepper steeped in hot water—or you can take a small capsule of cayenne powder (*Capsicum*, various species).

Consider learning a formal relaxation technique, such as tai chi, yoga, biofeedback, visualization, or meditation. While we now know that stress doesn't cause ulcers, we do know that stress can boost stomach acid production and worsen existing ulcers. "Your immune system is your body's way of taking care of viruses and bacteria. That system is damaged when it is repeatedly under stress," says J. Crit Harley, M.D., a behavioral medicine physician and director of Un-Limited Performance, a stress-management clinic in Hendersonville, North Carolina. "The ulcer is a sign that you are under stress, which can lower your immune status and allow bacteria to get a foothold. The opposite of the stress response is the relaxation response."

A licensed psychologist or behavioral medicine specialist—as well as numerous alternative healing practitioners—can teach you how to keep life's pressures from contributing to symptoms like ulcers. Relaxation techniques better prepare you for the next wave of negative events and give you more control, notes Dr. Harley.

Wrinkles

Years of exposure to sunlight or cigarette smoke can lead to wrinkles, as can decades of smiling, frowning, and squinting. All of these cause a breakdown in collagen, the intertwined cell layer that forms an elastic, spongy base under the second layer of skin. In your youth, collagen easily absorbs moisture and swells to keep your skin smooth and resilient. As you age, your body makes less collagen, and the existing collagen loses some of its ability to soak up water. Skin crevices that once formed a smooth terrain begin to collapse and fold, leaving wrinkles.

The Blended Prescription

Note: To learn about cautions and possible side effects of the remedies in this chapter, see page 253.

To repair already formed wrinkles, you can try various botanical remedies, and a dermatologist can prescribe a cream that will help stimulate collagen production. But wrinkle reversal isn't easy. The smart path is to avoid the things that promote wrinkles and do all you can to keep your skin moist and healthy. Here is a six-step prescription to achieve that, according to our blended-medicine experts.

It's simple but effective: Drink plenty of water, preferably eight 8-ounce glasses a day. Sure, skin is the outside layer of your body, but it gets most of its moisture from the bloodstream, not showers or baths. You need lots of water in your system to keep skin healthy and moist.

Each morning, after you clean your skin, rinse with lukewarm water, then apply a moisturizer to semi-wet skin. The goal with a moisturizer is to seal liquid in. If you first hydrate your skin with lukewarm water and just pat it dry, the moisturizer helps seal in that water.

Supplement with 1,000 to 2,000 milligrams of vitamin C a day. Vitamin C is an antioxidant that helps fight collagen breakdown, says Shiva Barton, N.D., a licensed acupuncturist and lead naturopathic physician at the Wellspace Health Center in Cambridge, Massachusetts. It slows the formation of wrinkles by helping to keep your collagen in a condition where it can retain moisture and "plump" the skin.

Each day, mix 1 tablespoon of flaxseed (*Linum usitatissimum*) oil into something you eat. Flaxseed oil has compounds that help keep your skin moist, says David Edelberg, M.D., assistant professor of medicine at Rush Medical College in Chicago and chairman and founder of the American WholeHealth Centers in Chicago, Boston, Denver, and Bethesda, Maryland. You can add it to cereal, pasta, or other foods that are part of your daily diet.

Put on sunscreen lotion whenever you spend time outdoors. Nothing breaks down collagen and ages skin as quickly and easily as the rays of the sun. Make sure the sunscreen you use has a sun protection factor (SPF) rating

HERBAL POWER

Rosy Skin

Evening primrose (*Oenothera biennis*) can help restore moisture to the skin, says David Edelberg, M.D., assistant professor of medicine at Rush Medical College in Chicago and chairman and founder of the American WholeHealth Centers in Chicago, Boston, Denver, and Bethesda, Maryland. Take one 1,000-milligram capsule of evening primrose oil twice daily, he suggests.

of 15 or higher and blocks out both types of ultraviolet rays, UVA and UVB, says Dee Anna Glaser, M.D., assistant professor of dermatology at St. Louis University School of Medicine in Missouri. Apply sunscreen 20 minutes before you head outside—yes, it takes that long to become effective—and reapply it every 1½ hours if you are swimming or participating in outdoor activities that make you sweat.

Cut back on cigarettes, caffeine, and alcohol. All three are toxins that can make your skin more prone to injury and damage. In addition, smoking causes blood vessels to constrict, which can starve skin of oxygen and nutrients. As for alcohol and caffeine, they, too, can make skin more susceptible to wrinkles since they cause dehydration.

Other Approaches

Slough off dead skin with a Buf-Puf once a day. Removing dead skin from your face helps make the living skin appear more supple, says Dr. Glaser. You can purchase a slightly rough cloth or Buf-Puf from a drugstore. Use it gently, with face soap and water. Your skin should never hurt when you use the puff.

Use a moisturizer that contains fruit acids. Fruit acids can help strengthen connective tissue, which makes your skin more resistant to wrinkles, Dr. Barton says. Fruit acids will be listed on the moisturizer's product label. Apply the moisturizer once or twice a day, he advises.

Ask your dermatologist about tretinoin emollient cream (Renova). Available by prescription, Renova helps stimulate collagen production so your skin looks more youthful, says Dr. Glaser. "Most of my patients seem really pleased with it." Follow your dermatologist's recommendations for applying it.

Consider acupuncture. Unlikely as it may seem, an acupuncture treatment applied directly to the crease of a wrinkle can help make the wrinkle disappear, according to Dr. Barton. This usually works best for people under 60, he says, and the full treatment sometimes involves 20 visits over the course of 10 weeks or so.

Yeast Infections

Normally, the vagina is a balanced ecosystem—a self-regulating, acidic environment with built-in safeguards against infection. Many microscopic organisms live there in harmony, including the "good" bacteria *Lactobacillus acidophilus*, which keep the environment acidic, and the yeastlike fungus *Candida albicans*. In a healthy vagina, these microorganisms compete for food, which prevents them from overpopulating. But when acidity in the vagina changes or when there is a higher-than-usual flow of estrogen, beneficial bacteria can die off, creating a nutrient-rich environment in which less benign yeast feast and thrive. While the yeast are happily reproducing, a woman can be driven nearly to distraction by the itching, burning, and discharge.

The Blended Prescription

Note: To learn about cautions and possible side effects of the remedies in this chapter, see page 253.

You can help prevent yeast infections by wearing loose-fitting pants and cotton underwear as well as avoiding vaginal deodorants, sprays, and douches.

If you think you have a yeast infection, a visit to the doctor is in order, just to make sure nothing else is wrong. Once your doctor has confirmed that you have this very familiar form of vaginitis, there are many possible solutions. Here are the top four recommendations of our blended-medicine experts, followed by several alternatives.

Try drugstore remedies first. Antifungal vaginal products like Gyne-Lotrimin and Monistat are highly effective; just follow the package instructions. "If a woman has been diagnosed once with a yeast infection and has the same symptoms, any over-the-counter antifungal is appropriate for self-treatment," says J. Christopher Carey, M.D., professor and vice chairman of the department of obstetrics and gynecology at Pennsylvania State University College of Medicine/Geisinger Health Systems in Hershey. You can choose a 1-, 3-, or 7-day treatment with either a cream or a suppository.

Swallow two 500-milligram capsules of the herb pau d'arco (*Tabebuia impetiginosa*) daily for 3 weeks. Pau d'arco is an antifungal that also boosts the immune system, says Cheri Annette Wagner, a member of the National Institute of Medical Herbalists and an herbalist at Equipoise

Center of America in Rochester, New York. If you prefer a tea, use 1 teaspoon of crushed pau d'arco bark to a cup of boiling water. Simmer, covered, for 10 to 15 minutes, then strain before drinking. Have three to six cups daily for 3 weeks, even after your symptoms are gone, she says.

Make a douche of *Lactobacillus acidophilus*. Mix enough acidophilus powder (or enough capsule con-

---

HERBAL POWER

Anti-Yeast Rescue Tea

Here is an effective traditional herbal blend to ease the misery of yeast infections and prevent them from paying a repeat visit, says Cheri Annette Wagner, a member of the National Institute of Medical Herbalists and an herbalist at Equipoise Center of America in Rochester, New York. Combine the following herbs.

Echinacea (Echinacea purpurea): 3 tablespoons, to strengthen immunity

Calendula (Calendula officinalis): 3 tablespoons, for its antifungal properties

Licorice (Glycyrrhiza glabra): 1 to 2 tablespoons, for its anti-inflammatory powers

Stinging nettle (Urtica dioica): 3 tablespoons, for its calcium and other nutritives as well as chlorophyll, which helps to build healthy, mineral-rich blood

Verbena (Verbena officinalis): 3 tablespoons, to stabilize blood sugar during a time when you might be cutting back on sugar and carbohydrates

Steep all these herbs in a quart of hot water for 10 to 15 minutes, then strain before drinking. You can drink up to six cups a day for the most healing effect, says Wagner.

tents) into ¼ cup of warm water to provide 10 billion organisms. Then, using an empty douche bag, douche the mixture into the vagina once a day for no more than 2 weeks. Or mix 1 cup of yogurt containing live cultures with 1 cup of warm water. Douche with the mixture three times a week until symptoms are gone. Be careful: Excessive douching can upset the natural habitat of the vagina. If you're pregnant, consult with your physician before douching.

For yeast infections that keep coming back despite treatment, ask your doctor about fluconazole (Diflucan). This powerful prescription antifungal medicine clears up yeast infections in one dose, says Dr. Carey.

Other Approaches

Make an antiseptic suppository by filling a number 3 gelatin capsule with 500 milligrams of powdered boric acid. "Boric acid is great for treating fungal infections that resist over-the-counter medications," says Dr. Carey. Simply insert the filled capsule into your vagina once daily for 10 to 14 days, he says. If you want to try this treatment, make sure to inform your doctor first.

Chop one to three cloves of fresh, raw garlic and mix it into your foods throughout the day while you are having acute symptoms and for a week afterward. Garlic contains allicin and other components that are powerful antifungal and antibacterial agents, Wagner says. If you can't stand the taste or odor of fresh garlic, look for odorless garlic capsules. Take 900 to 1,500 milligrams daily through at least a week after your symptoms are gone, she says.

Sponge relief with oatmeal. Fill the foot of an old (but clean) pair of nylons with a cup of loose oatmeal, says Dr.

Carey. Then seal it with a rubber band. Run a warm bath, letting the oatmeal "sponge" steep in the water like a tea bag. Relax in the tub for 10 to 15 minutes. Then use the oatmeal sponge to gently swab the external area of your vagina and rinse with clean water. Oatmeal soothes and relieves irritated skin. Yeast love a moist environment, so be sure to dry off thoroughly after bathing. Take care when stepping out of the tub; oatmeal can make the surface slick.

For 10 minutes, apply a washcloth soaked in witch hazel. Witch hazel casts a soothing spell, shrinking inflamed tissue and relieving itching and burning. You can either soak a washcloth with witch hazel or buy presoaked pads (like Tucks), says Dr. Carey. The witch hazel will be especially soothing if you cool it in the refrigerator before using it, he notes.

To add healing power, put 10 drops of antifungal tea tree (*Melaleuca alternifolia*) oil or calendula (*Calendula officinalis*) oil in a cup of witch hazel, says Wagner. Apply it as directed above.

Dry the vaginal area thoroughly when finished with either witch hazel treatment.

Apply an herbal salve. Mix 4 ounces of aloe vera gel with 25 drops of essential oils of marjoram (*Origanum onites*), lavender (*Lavandula angustifolia*), or calendula (*Calendula officinalis*) and apply to the outside area of the vagina in the morning and the evening for a week. This cooling salve soothes the burning and itching you feel during the acute phase of yeast infections, says Wagner. And marjoram, lavender, and calendula are all infection-fighting herbs, she adds. Make sure to wash your hands with soap and water before and after applying.

Prepare an herbal wash with tinctures of calendula (*Calendula officinalis*) and myrrh (*Commiphora molmol*). Both have antifungal properties, and calendula strengthens your body's own ability to prevent infection, says Wagner. Stir 5 to 10 drops of each tincture into 8 ounces of clean filtered water. Use a clean douche bag to rinse the outer area of your vagina once a day for 5 minutes or until the bag is empty. Use this herbal wash for up to 3 weeks, she says.

Swallow one 100-milligram capsule or 10 to 12 drops of grapefruit seed extract in 6 ounces of water three times daily for up to 3 weeks. Grapefruit seed extract helps destroy the yeast while helping to replenish healthy bacteria, says Wagner.

Using Self-Care Safely

The prescriptions presented in this book combine the best conventional and alternative therapies to quickly relieve symptoms and speed healing. To get the most benefit from the individual remedies, you need to know how to use them correctly and safely.

Below, you will find dosage recommendations, contraindications, potential side effects, and other essential information about specific remedies. This information is based on advice from health care professionals who have worked extensively with these remedies as well as on guidelines from authoritative references, such as the *American Herbal Products Association's Botanical Safety Handbook, Homeopathy: The Principles and Practice of Treatment,* and *The Illustrated Encyclopedia of Essential Oils.*

Remember, a remedy is most effective when used properly. So check here before beginning self-care. If you have been diagnosed with a chronic health condition or if you take prescription drugs regularly and want to use any of the remedies mentioned in this book, talk with your health care practitioner first.

Women who are pregnant or nursing or who are trying to become pregnant should always consult their doctors before using any home remedy—including vitamins, herbs, essential oils, and homeopathic remedies—or taking a prescription or over-the-counter medication. And none of these remedies should be used with infants or small children without a doctor's supervision.

Potential Side Effects and Guidelines for Safe Use of Remedies

Acetaminophen Consult your doctor before using if you have kidney or liver damage.

Acupressure (general) Avoid pressure that is uncomfortable. If you have questions about or problems with technique, consult an acupressure professional, such as a licensed acupuncturist or a licensed massage therapist.

Aloe In gel form, may delay wound healing; do not use externally on any surgical incision. Do not ingest the dried leaf, as it is a habit-forming laxative.

Arnica Do not apply to broken skin. Avoid contact with the eyes.

Aspirin Do not use if you have asthma or chronic stomach problems, unless instructed by your physician.

Black cohosh Do not use for more than 6 months.

Bromelain May cause nausea, vomiting, diarrhea, skin rash, and heavy menstrual bleeding. May increase the risk of bleeding in people taking aspirin or anticoagulants (blood thinners). Do not use if allergic to pineapple.

Bruise plaster Discontinue use if skin becomes irritated.

Calcium Consult your doctor before taking more than 2,500 milligrams a day.

Capsaicin Do not use cream for more than 2 consecutive days; wait 14 days before resuming treatment. Discontinue using if skin becomes irritated. Avoid contact with the eyes and injured skin.

Cascara sagrada Do not use if you have any inflammatory condition of the intestines, intestinal obstruction, or abdominal pain. Can cause laxative dependency and diarrhea. Do not use for more than 14 days.

Cat's claw Do not use if you have hemophilia. Side effects may include headache, stomachache, or difficulty breathing.

Cayenne Do not use externally near eyes or on injured skin. May cause gastrointestinal irritation when taken internally on an empty stomach.

Chamomile Very rarely, can cause an allergic reaction when ingested. People allergic to closely related plants, such as ragweed, asters, and chrysanthemums, should drink the tea with caution.

Chasteberry May counteract the effectiveness of birth control pills.

Chromium picolinate Consult your doctor before taking more than 200 micrograms a day.

Cinnamon Do not use the aromatic oil for more than 2 weeks without the guidance of a qualified practitioner.

Copper Consult your doctor before taking more than 10 milligrams a day; smaller doses, taken occasionally, are considered safe.

Dandelion root Consult your doctor before using if you have gallbladder disease.

Devil's claw Do not use if you have gastric or duodenal ulcers. Consult your physician before using if you have gallstones.

Dimenhydrinate (Dramamine) May cause drowsiness, dizziness, blurred vision, or dry mouth.

Echinacea Do not use if allergic to closely related plants such as ragweed, asters, and chrysanthemums. Do not use if you have tuberculosis or an autoimmune condition, such as multiple sclerosis or lupus, because echinacea stimulates the immune system.

Essential oils (general) With few exceptions, essential oils are not taken internally. Avoid contact with the eyes. If essential oils come in contact with the eyes, flush immediately with cold water. Consult a physician if irritation or inflammation persists. Don't apply essential oils undiluted. Dilute them in a carrier base, which can be an oil (such as almond), cream, or gel, before application. Many essential oils can cause skin irritation or allergic reactions in people with sensitive skin. Before applying any new oil to the skin, always do a patch test: Put a few drops on the back of your wrist. Wait for an hour or more. If irritation or redness occurs, wash the area with cold water, and, in the future, avoid the oil altogether. Do not use essential oils at home for serious medical or psychological problems. Store essential oils in dark bottles, away from heat and light and out of the reach of children and pets.

Eucalyptus Doses of the herb exceeding 4 grams a day may cause nausea, vomiting, and diarrhea. Do not use if you have severe liver disease or an inflammatory disease of the bile ducts or gastrointestinal tract. Do not use the essential oil for more than 2 weeks without the guidance of a qualified practitioner. Do not use more than three drops in the bath. Do not use at the same time as homeopathic remedies.

Feverfew If chewed, fresh leaves can cause mouth sores in some people.

Fish oil Increases bleeding time, possibly resulting in nosebleeds, and may cause easy bruising and stomach upset. Do not use if you have a bleeding disorder, have uncontrolled high blood pressure, are taking anticoagulants (blood thinners), use aspirin regularly, or are allergic to any kind of fish. Take fish oil, not fish-liver oil, which is high in vitamins A and D and can be toxic in high amounts. People with diabetes should not take fish oil because of its high fat content.

Folic acid Doses above 1,000 micrograms must be taken under medical supervision. Do not use without the guidance of a trained practitioner if you have anemia.

Garlic Do not use supplements if you are on anticoagulants (blood thinners) or before undergoing surgery, because garlic thins the blood and may increase bleeding. Do not use if you're taking drugs to lower your blood sugar. Do not use the essential oil in your ear if you have a perforated eardrum. Do not use more than three drops in the bath.

Ginger May increase bile secretion, so if you have gallstones, do not use therapeutic amounts of the dried root or powder without guidance from a health care practitioner. Fresh ginger is safe when used to season food.

Ginkgo Do not use with antidepressant MAO inhibitor drugs such as phenelzine sulfate (Nardil) or tranylcypromine (Parnate), aspirin or other nonsteroidal anti-inflammatory medications, or blood-thinning medications such as warfarin (Coumadin). Can cause dermatitis, diarrhea, and vomiting in doses higher than 240 milligrams of concentrated extract.

Ginseng May cause irritability if taken with caffeine or other stimulants. Do not use if you have high blood pressure.

Globe artichoke May cause a reaction in people who are allergic to other plants in the daisy family, such as chamomile and marigold.

Goldenseal Do not use if you have high blood pressure.

Guar gum May interfere with the absorption of certain nutrients and medications. Do not use if you have a bowel obstruction. Take with at least 8 ounces of water.

Homeopathic remedies (general) May become less potent with caffeine consumption. Homeopathic treatment is not compatible with black pepper, camphor, eucalyptus, and peppermint.

Hops Rarely, can cause skin rash, so handle fresh or dried hops carefully. Do not use if you are prone to or have depression.

Horse chestnut May interfere with the action of other drugs, especially blood thinners such as warfarin (Coumadin). May irritate the gastrointestinal tract.

Horsetail May cause thiamin deficiency. Do not use tincture if you have heart or kidney problems. Do not take more than 2 grams per day of powdered extract or take for prolonged periods.

Hydroxycitric acid Do not use if you have severe liver or kidney disease. May cause gastrointestinal irritation if you have an ulcer.

Hyssop Do not use the essential oil for more than 2 weeks without the guidance of a qualified practitioner. Do not use if you have high blood pressure. Do not use if you have epilepsy.

Ibuprofen Do not take if you have asthma or chronic stomach problems, unless directed by your physician.

Juniper Do not use the essential oil for more than 2 weeks without the guidance of a qualified practitioner. Do not use if you have kidney disease.

Kaffir potato May lower blood pressure; consult your doctor before using if you are taking high blood pressure or asthma medications. Do not use if you have ulcers.

Kava kava Do not take with alcohol or barbiturates. Do not take more than the recommended dose on the package. Use caution when driving or operating equipment, since this herb is a muscle relaxant.

Lemon Do not use more than three drops in the bath. Avoid direct sunlight, because this oil can cause skin sensitivity.

Licorice Do not use for more than 4 to 6 weeks, because overuse can lead to water retention, high blood pressure caused by potassium loss, or impaired heart or kidney function. Do not use if you have diabetes, high blood pressure, a liver or kidney disorder, or low potassium.

Magnesium May cause diarrhea. Consult your doctor before using if you have a heart or kidney problem.

Ma huang (ephedra) Use only under the guidance of a qualified practitioner.

Melatonin Take no more than 1 milligram daily. It causes drowsiness, so take only at bedtime; never take before driving. Do not use if you have an autoimmune disease such as rheumatoid arthritis or lupus or a personal or family history of a hormone-dependent cancer such as breast, testicular, prostate, or endometrial. Consult your doctor before using if you are on a prescription medication. Interactions, though rare, do occur. May cause headache, morning dizziness, daytime sleepiness, depression, and upset stomach.

Mullein Do not use the essential oil in your ear if you have a perforated eardrum.

Myrrh Can irritate the kidneys and cause diarrhea. Do not use if you have uterine bleeding.

Niacin Doses exceeding 35 milligrams a day require medical supervision.

Peppermint Do not use more than three drops of the essential oil in the bath. Do not use at the same time as homeopathic remedies. Ingestion of peppermint essential oil may lead to stomach upset in sensitive individuals. If you have gallbladder or liver disease, do not use without medical supervision.

Psyllium Do not use if you have a bowel obstruction. Take 1 hour after other drugs. Take with at least 8 ounces of water.

Rhus toxicodendron Consult your doctor if your pain persists or worsens, if you notice redness or swelling, or if new symptoms develop.

Rosemary May cause excessive menstrual bleeding in therapeutic amounts. Considered safe when used as a spice. Do not use the essential oil if you have high blood pressure or epilepsy.

St. John's wort Do not use with antidepressants without medical approval. May cause photosensitivity; avoid overexposure to direct sunlight.

Saw palmetto Consult your doctor if using to treat an enlarged prostate.

Stinging nettle If you have allergies, your symptoms may worsen, so take only one dose a day for the first few days.

Traumed ointment For external use only. Do not apply to broken skin or open wounds.

Turmeric Do not use as a home remedy if you have high stomach acid, ulcers, gallstones, or a bile duct obstruction. Safe to use as a seasoning on food.

Valerian Do not use with sleep-enhancing or mood-regulating medication, because it may intensify their effects. Discontinue if stimulant action (nervousness or heart palpitation) occurs.

Vitamin A Do not take more than 10,000 international units a day unless directed by your doctor. Because of the risk of birth defects, pregnant women should avoid doses of 5,000 IU or more.

Vitamin B$_6$ Doses above 100 milligrams must be taken under medical supervision.

Vitamin C May cause diarrhea when taken in doses of more than 1,000 milligrams a day. Supplements made from a corn base may cause a reaction in people who are allergic to corn.

Vitamin E Consult your doctor before taking more than 400 international units a day; one study using low-dose supplementation showed increased risk of hemorrhagic stroke.

Willow Do not use if you need to avoid aspirin, especially if you are taking blood-thinning medication such as warfarin (Coumadin), because its active ingredient is related to aspirin. May interact with barbiturates or sedatives such as aprobarbital (Amytal) or alprazolam (Xanax). Can cause stomach irritation when consumed with alcohol. Do not give to children under age 16 who have fever or viral infections, including chicken pox or the flu; may contribute to Reye's syndrome, which affects the brain and liver.

Yarrow Handling flowers can cause skin rash in rare cases.

Zinc Do not exceed 20 milligrams a day unless directed by your physician.

Zinc gluconate lozenges May cause nausea, so take immediately after meals. Avoid lozenges containing citrate, tartrate, orotate, or mannitol/sorbitol; these substances diminish potency. Discontinue use after 1 week.

Zinc solution spray Avoid contact with the eyes.

Index

Underscored page references indicate boxed text.